Thank you to my husband Ross, for his love and support in helping me to collect the necessary photographs, in a one-day marathon at Chelsea; thank you also to Brooke, our graphic designer, who works her magic in making the books ready for printing, and to Paul, our web technician who also works his magic in keeping the websites active and responsive.

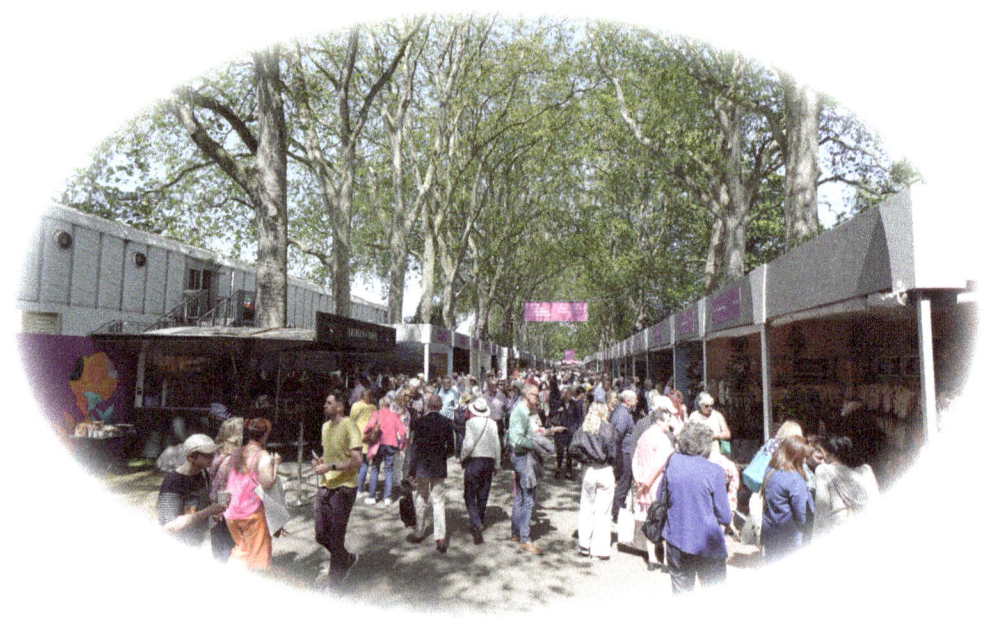

Welcome to Part One –

'The Magic of Chelsea' -
A Flower Show Like No Other

It is great to have so many people enjoying our latest 'Magic of Chelsea' book. With so many people worldwide unable to get to the magnificent flower displays and the other features of the show, it is our joy and privilege to bring the first part of the book to you.

We have decided to split the book into three, which allows people to collect the books at the time they are ready for the next part of our yearly adventure.

During the visit, we collect many photographs, possibly a thousand or more, and sadly, we have to leave many photographs out of the book, because simply, we do not have enough pages to show them all.

We have a lot of fun working on this book and we know you will enjoy the books as we do in creating them.

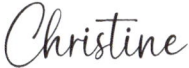

It's 2023 and there we were, waiting at the station to catch the train into Paddington, London, and then, we travelled on the underground train to Sloane Street, Station…

The excitement was mounting as many people started to leave the train for the walk to the Chelsea Flower Show.

There he was, a man in a brightly coloured shirt offering lifts in his rikshaw, the opportunity to ride through London in this way was too great to pass up and the ride was excellent, seeing sights often taken for granted when in the car…!

At the gate, where many people patiently waited, the day had begun and what a day we had in the beautiful spring sun…

Please see the following pages to follow our journey and the beauty of a magnificent flower show –

The Magic of Chelsea

The Respect They Deserve...

Isn't about time we gave the respect back to our native insects, their environments, and homes?

For well over two hundred years our insects have been in their personal fight to survive. They don't have a voice, they cannot shout, scream, and make a noise when their homes are destroyed, the only sign they give, is when they no longer exist...!

The emphasis for the 2023 Chelsea Flower Show was on native fields and meadow flowers and grasses, and how refreshing to see the abundance of differently coloured flowers, their shape, form, texture, and vibrancy; some petals glistened as the rays of sunshine caught their movement in the soft spring breeze, and what a treat for any human being to enjoy the moments of this year's Chelsea Flower Show...!

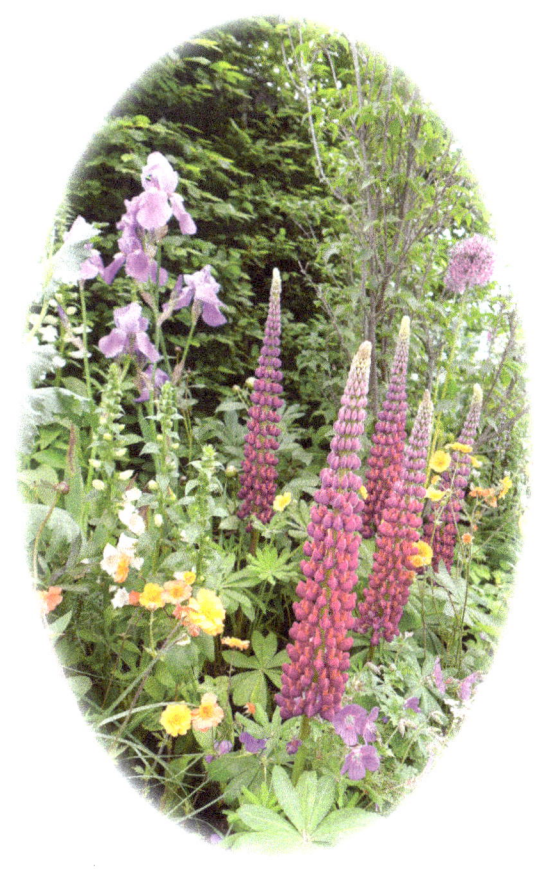

They Want to Survive...

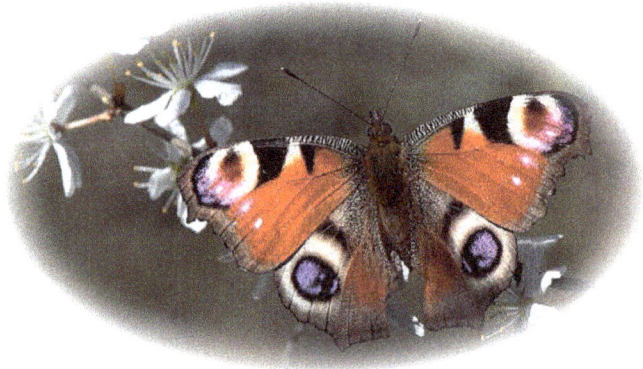

The butterfly you see, has many jobs to do, not only the will to survive but to pollenate the flowers it visits but to make babies for next year too…!

Its time spent is only a few, with so many jobs, and soon, this beautiful creature will need to support the new…

So fragile its wings and glorious too, but delicate as fairy dust, and now too often, too few…!

The butterfly has many messages to give, for it is the story, the story to live…!

Like mothers, from nature we find, the will to produce their babies each year, and to do just that, they need to know the earth will be kind…!

For once the babies are new, the mum's job is done, its short life is lived, for its legacy it leaves, its babies for next year, the flowers it pollinates and the beauty it gives…!

When you see your next butterfly, please take the time to ponder, and then wonder, not only at the joy of the sight, but at the work it does with all its might….!

If you have purchased this book without its cover, it may be a stolen book.

Neither the publisher or the author is under any obligation to provide professional services in anyway, legal, health or in any form which is related to this book, its contents advice or otherwise.

The law and practices vary from country to country and state to state.

If legal or professional information is required, the purchaser, or the reader should seek the information privately and best suited to their particular needs, and circumstances.

The author and publisher specifically disclaim any liability that may be incurred from the information within this book.

All rights reserved. No part of this book, including the interior design, images, cover design, diagrams, or any intellectual property (IP), icons and photographs may be reproduced or transmitted in any form by any means (electronic, photocopying, recording or otherwise) without the prior permission of the publisher. ©

Copyright© 2023 MSI Australia

All rights reserved.

ISBN: 978-0-6459403-6-7

Published by How2Books
Under licence from MSI Ltd, Australia
Company Registration No: 96963518255
NSW, Australia

See our website: www.how2books.com.au
Or contact by email: sales@how2books.com.au
Covers and Copyright owned by MSI, Australia

MSI acknowledges the author and images, text and photographs used in this book.

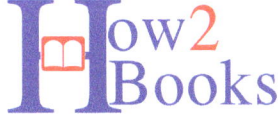

10% of the sale of each book helps to support Diabetes Type One and Cancer Research.

The Back Story

Six O'clock on the dot, the taxi arrives! The early autumn morning in Australia is beautiful in April with a slight change in the colour of the leaves on the trees, as they turn from green to slight gold. From the drop off at the station in Bowral, New South Wales, and as we sit on the train on the way to Sydney Airport, it's time to inhale, take a deep breath, and the time to think about the journey we've just begun...

With so many kilometres to travel, there is no time to stop, the hustle and bustle of the time, keeps us alert and ready to go at a 'drop of a hat!' Trains, airports, rental cars, all with many people making their way to different worldwide destinations!

Most faces are concerning with the look, 'I hope this is the right way to go, or is this the flight we take...?' And so it is, the long-haul from one side of the planet to the other...! Regardless of lengthy waits, airport crowds and long-distance travel, how many generations have had the privilege of flying across the oceans, baron areas of land below, and still be served food on the flight and a glass or two of wine or a coffee when needed...?

The technology needed to bring our books to our readers is mesmerizing and yet, we use it without much thought. Once my brain accepts, we are living in the here and now, the flight journey has come to an end, and we are there in the Baggage Hall at Heathrow Airport...

It's amazing how the scramble, each person goes through, to collect their bags and it never seems to change! We have waited for bags, that don't appear because they have been left at an airport in Australia...! We have also been fortunate enough to have the bags come around on the first baggage carousel to circulate...! The bags collected; we make our way to the hire car. and what a relief to finally sit in the passenger seat and, at last, to see the different greens on the forming leaf buds as they show their many different greens. Just one sunny day was needed to bring the trees of the South of England into magnificent colour. Alas, it was too cold to allow that to happen...!

It was the 14th of April, we were there, at the 15th Century Notley Abbey, and to see our beautiful Goddaughter married. The weather was cold and wet, but the bride was radiant and gorgeous. Many weeks pass and we are on the train heading to The Chelsea Flower Show. Memories rush into my head, how the time has flown since I did my training in London to become a florist, and yet my heart and mind long for the colours, textures, and vibrancy of the flowers I will later see that day!

I'm jolted into the current moment, we are there, at Sloane Street, Station, and the crowds start to stand up from their train seats and want to step out onto the platform. Though there are many people, order is a priority for the excited crowd. No grim faces could be seen, just people happy to enjoy the moments of the day!

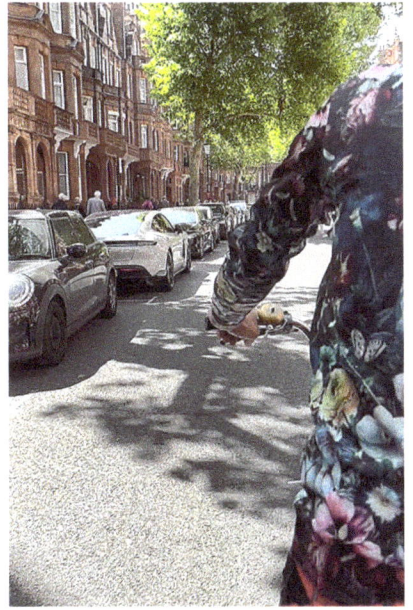

Emerging into the bright sunlight from the darkness of the station, my eyes were transfixed on a man wearing a brightly coloured floral shirt; he was the rikshaw driver and I was determined to make the most of the day, I persuaded my husband to part with, what was meant to be a fifteen-pound ride into a twenty-pound ride…, at the end of the trip…!

It was wonderful to see these parts of London, not normally seen when we are looking for parking or on a busy London bus!

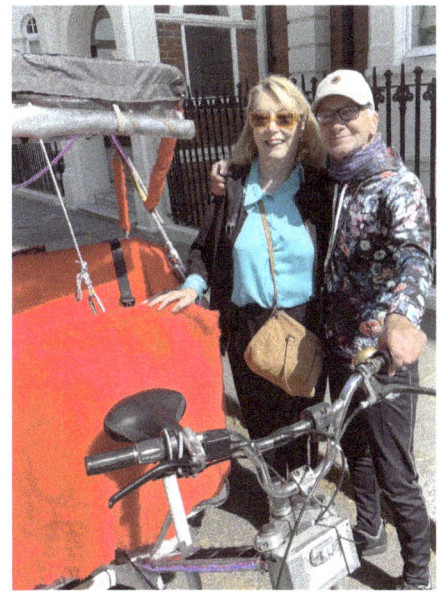

As we travelled on our short journey to the flower show, I couldn't help thinking about my own studies, not only as a florist in London, but one amazing year spent at the Canberra School of Art where I studied 20th century art history and sculpting. These studies have brought together the knowledge I now have in the ability to make meaningful comments about the exhibits on display in 2023.

Now, to our readers, please enjoy this lovely new edition of 'The Magic of Chelsea'.

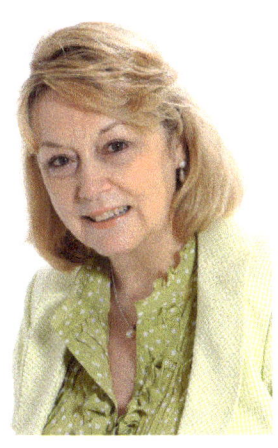

Christine

Christine Thompson-Wells, Author of Many Books
CEO, How2Books &
Full Potential Education & Training
BA Education, Dip of Teaching, MACEA,
CPD Accredited Education

Content   Page

The Reason Why…?	1
The Reason Why – Poem	2
People On the Move	3
The Clematis as it Grows	4
Clematis – Poem	5
Sculpture	6
Sculpture – Mesmerizing Creations	7
Gentle Thoughts of Childhood	9
A Time to Think and Take a Moment – Poem	11
The Inspiration of Shape	12
From Flowing Form to the Movement of Glass – A Combination of Glass and Steel	15
With Impression – The Merging of Water and Sculpture	17
Paul Richardson	19
From the Rock it Comes – Poem	20
From Rock	21
James Parker – Sculpture	23
Light in the Garden	25
A Day of Fun	27
The Art of Floristry Design	28
The Art of Floristry Design…	29
Floristry and Floral Art	43
The Floris – Poem	44
The Mush Room	47
The Mush Room…	48
Shapes, Colour & Texture	50

The Reason Why...?

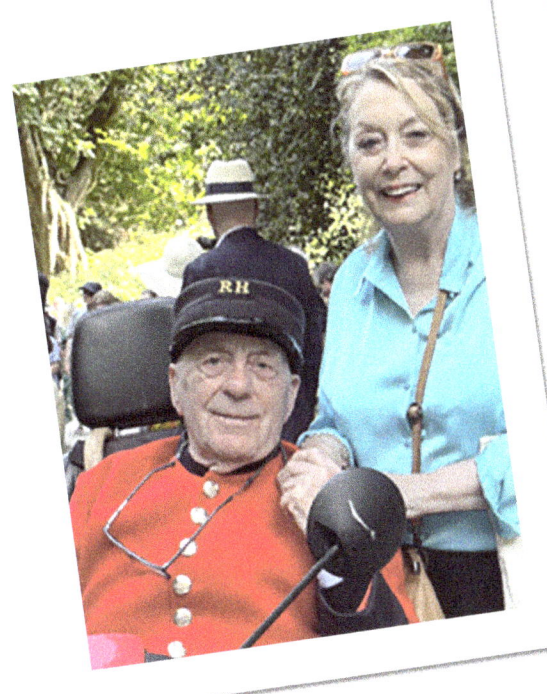

Since 1804, the RHS Chelsea Flower Show, has been an annual event. Originally it was called The Great Spring Show.

In 1913, it was moved to its present location at the Royal Hospital, Chelsea.

It's the glamour and excitement that makes the flower show such an exciting event. It is the event in many people's calendars each year that allows the show to be the success it is in the twenty-first century.

The Royal Hospital, Chelsea, is home to about three hundred British Army veterans, which include both men and women, all of which call the hospital, 'Home'.

Many of the veterans have served in Cyprus, Northern Ireland, the Falklands War, and the Second World War, from (1939-1945).

Originally, and the precursor to the establishment of the hospital in 1677, it was established for officers of disbanded regiments, soldiers with injuries, which was the original force by Sir Stephen Fox (1627-1716). Royal patronage was added to the establishment by King Charles II in 1682. The purpose of the hospital was to establish a retreat for war veterans.

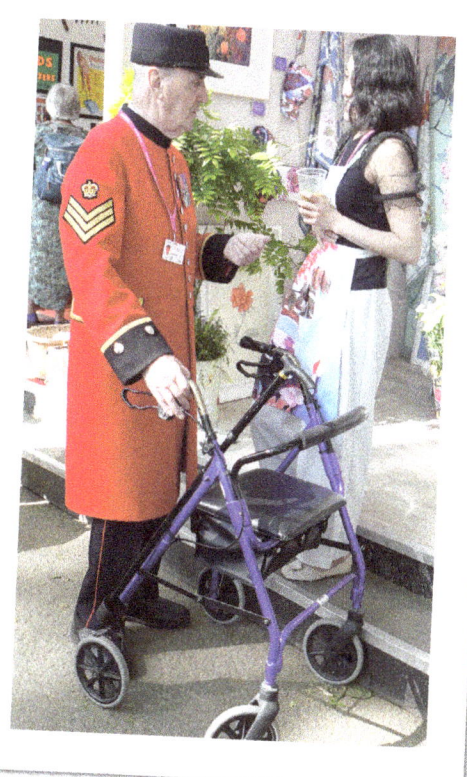

The Reason Why...?

So many times, we see, the people that have served…
To keep our lands free…!

Through years of battle, we are here, not by chance you know, but by dedication of the people we cannot see…!

The numbers too great to count, but sometimes we may reflect, on those past lives that allow us to live our daily lives…
Though they may be humble, we are at least free…!

With the tradition we hold, those lives once lived, and may we not forget the enormous price they paid…!

To allow us to make the choices we freely make as from day to day
We learn….

The wonders of the moments, some of the past veterans did not have time to yearn…!

For this is the reason, that so many can enjoy, the wonders of the Chelsea Show that so many have not had the time to know…!

Many people want to see the wonders of the show, and yet, it's time to stop, reflect, and the Reason Why we know….!

In Remembrance.

People on the Move
The Enjoyment of the day...

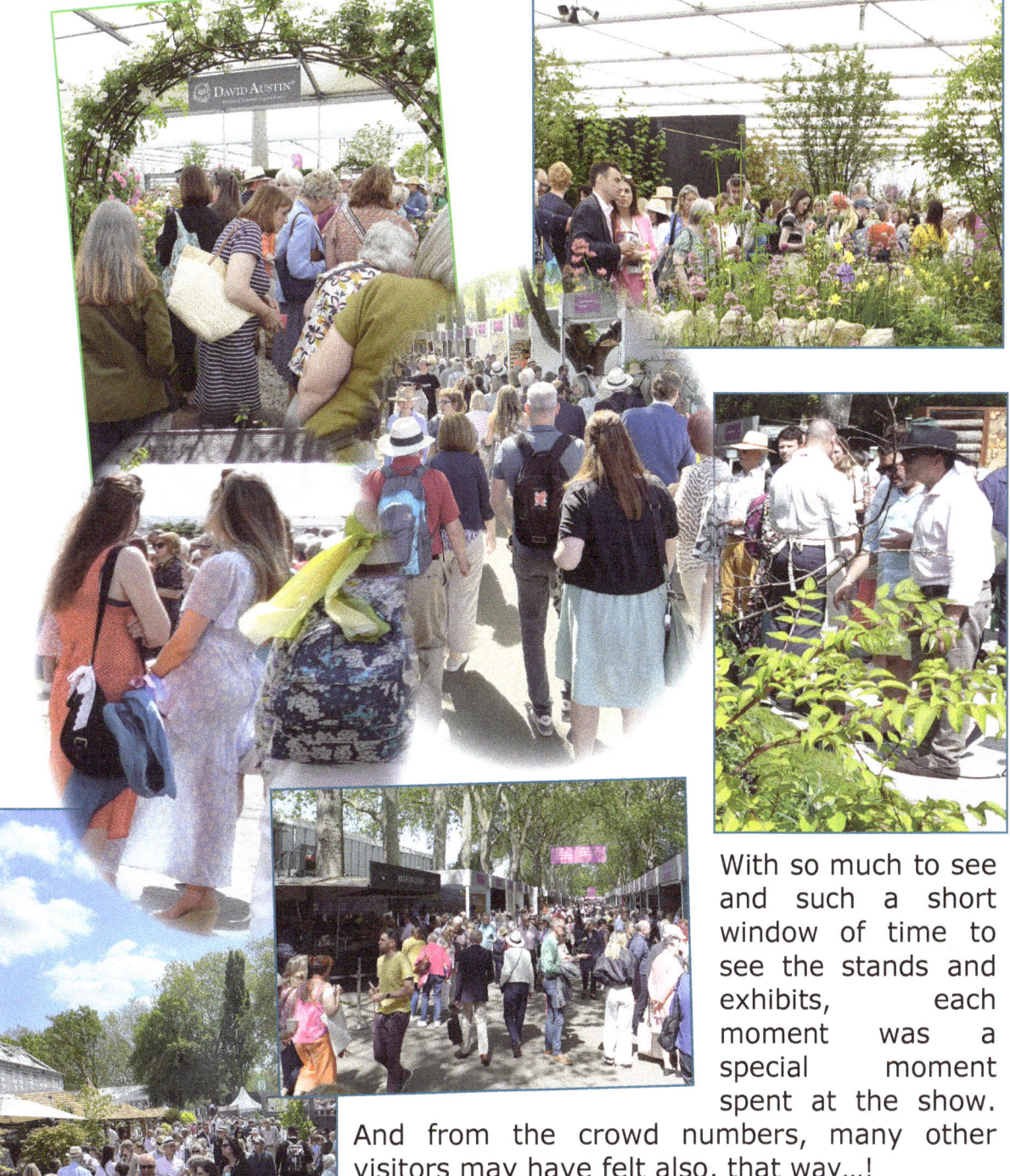

With so much to see and such a short window of time to see the stands and exhibits, each moment was a special moment spent at the show. And from the crowd numbers, many other visitors may have felt also, that way...!

The Clematis as it Grows

The clematis is such an extraordinary flower; it has a delicate and petal combination that holds your vision as you look deeply into the flower's centre.

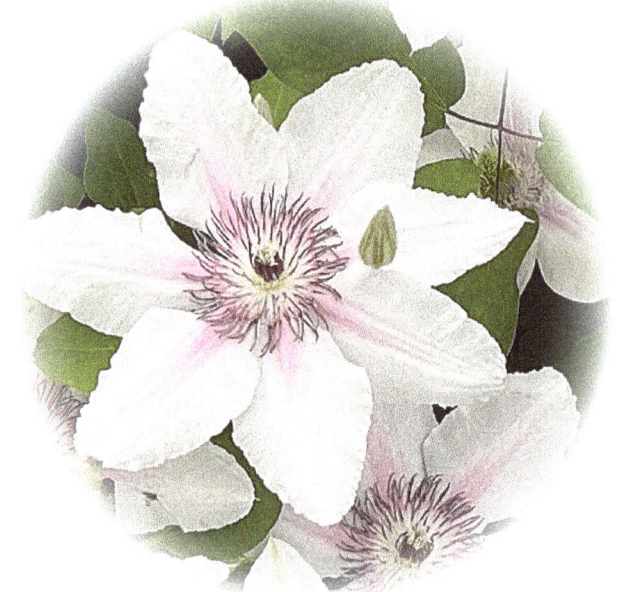

In this beautiful photograph, the gentle pink hue, with a slight hint of deep maroon towards the ovary of the flower shows this beauty.

Gentle petals shown, show soft the white outer petals leading the eye through the deeper pink and veins of the petal, which all lead to the magnificent centre of filaments and anthers, such a beautiful combination of
colour it also makes one think of the porcelain china once used for afternoon teas and of years gone by…!

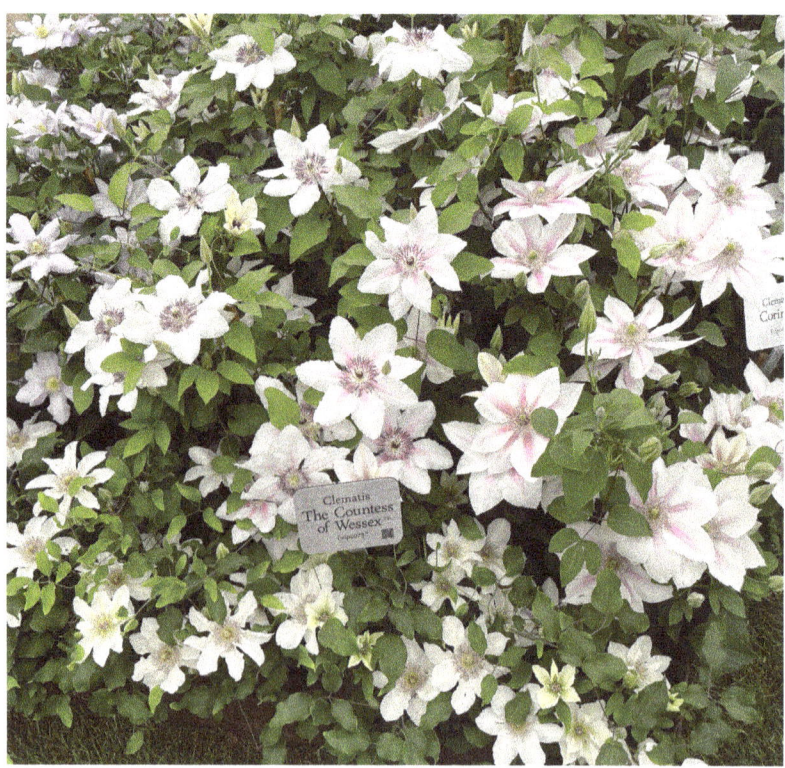

This new cultivar named the Duchess of Wessex displayed a magnificent show of such fine flowers.

This variety had a soft, but delicious scent and created a soothing combination within such a busy location.

Clematis come in many colours from purples to soft pinks and stunning whites. Most develop a woody type of stem as they mature.

Clematis

She holds her head in wonder as she flirts within the show…!

With many colours she flaunts, and just to let us know…!
Many single flowers to display, and hold our vision so, and as we gasp and say 'show some more…'
Our hearts will gently soar…!

The mischief she holds so dear, is part of her lasting charm…
For within such beauty, there cannot be any harm….!

As new petals unfurl and old flowers wither in the sun…
The short and beauty of the day is speckled with great fun…!

For porcelain the petals seem on appearance as you look, but beyond the delicate structure is the story within the book…!

Like so many flowers before her grew…
and so beautiful, and alas, only now, it is too few…!

The clematis, as we see it in the show, and what a sight…
for those simple petals will fade throughout the night…!

And it is with memories we linger of a spectacle once seen…
The clematis is recharging for the show she was so keen…!

And for next year she flowers again and the beauty to behold
for the beauty within this flower is magnificent and bold…!

Sculpture

With many creative displays in this year's show, it is difficult to identify a favourite! We apologise, if we have missed your designs, but we can only offer so much space within our book.

The ideas within the sculptures that follow, were major talking points, and points of inspiration, not only for the show visitors, but we are sure, for the creators of the masterpieces.

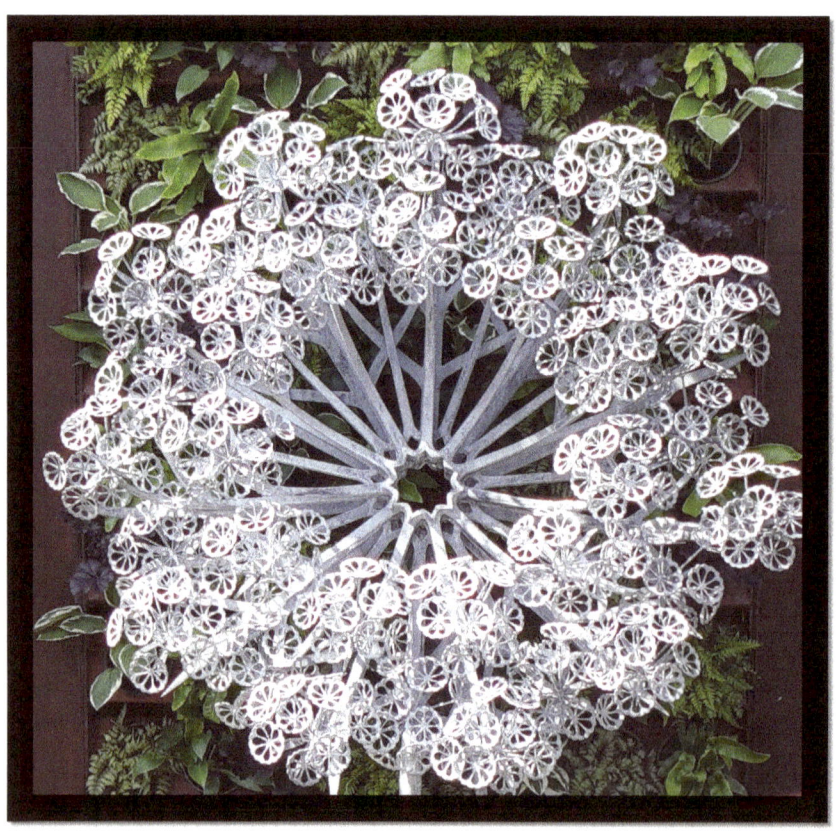

Sculpture – Mezmerising Creations

The show did not miss out on presenting many amazing sculptures this year, with many representations, show the beauty of the planet and the birds that fly the skies.

Opposite, mezmerising shapes, all giving their own version of our planet and the flight of the swallows.

Swallows travel many thousands of miles and arrive in the United Kingdom, from Africa, in April each year. They are ready to make their return journey by about September.

A delightful sculpture gives us the story of the swallows' flight...!

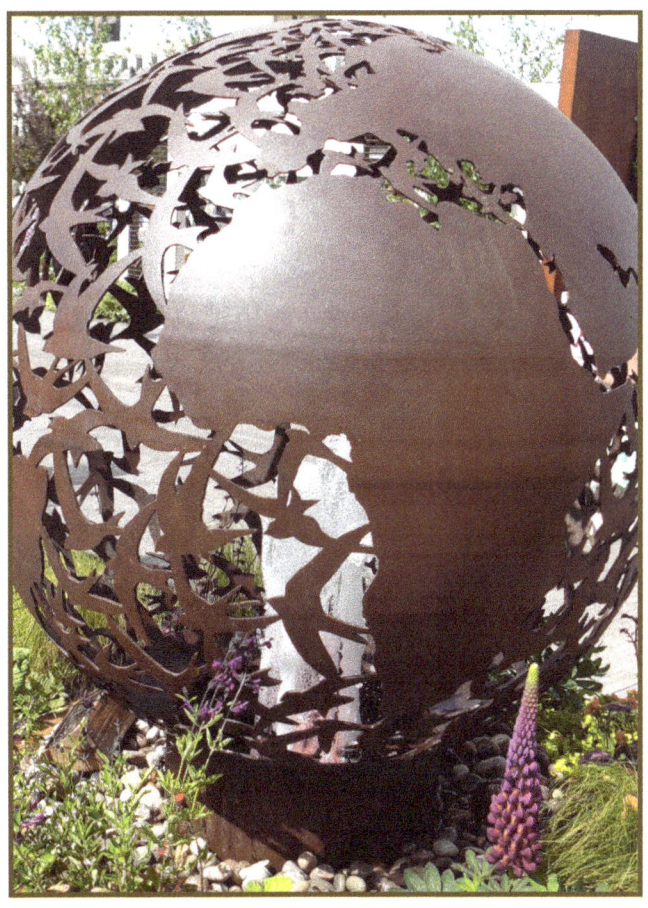

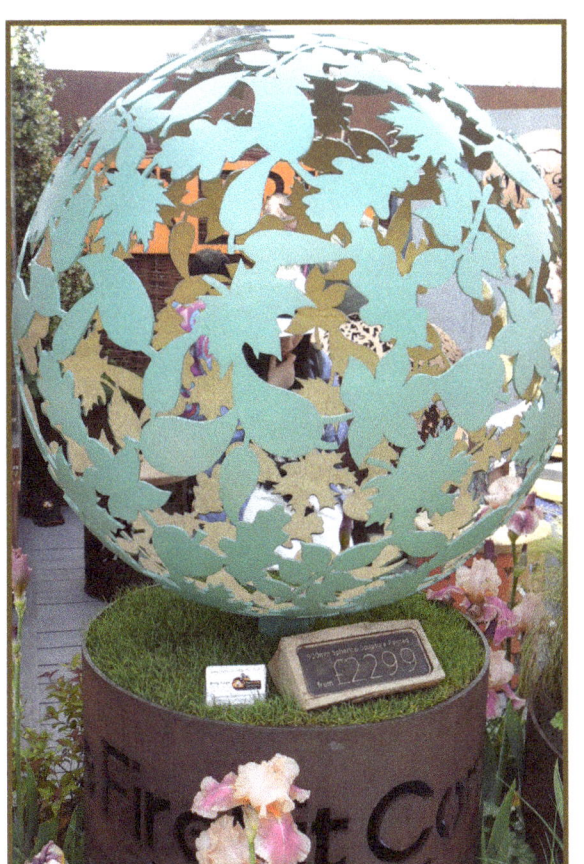

Considering we had a luggage weight we needed to think about, it would be nice to just slip one of these magnificent sculptures into the handbag, but alas, too big for such a thought or consideration...!

Opposite, the aqua colour of cut leaf shapes allows you to wonder and yet the softness of the colour, is, restful for the eye...!

To keep the orb or globe shape so perfectly balanced, round, and yet, to give the appearance of almost a lace of iron or steel work, within the sculpture, allows us to think about the gentleness of the force within the materials used in this display.

In the below sculpture, the added use of water creates a gentle flow of movement, and softness of sound....!

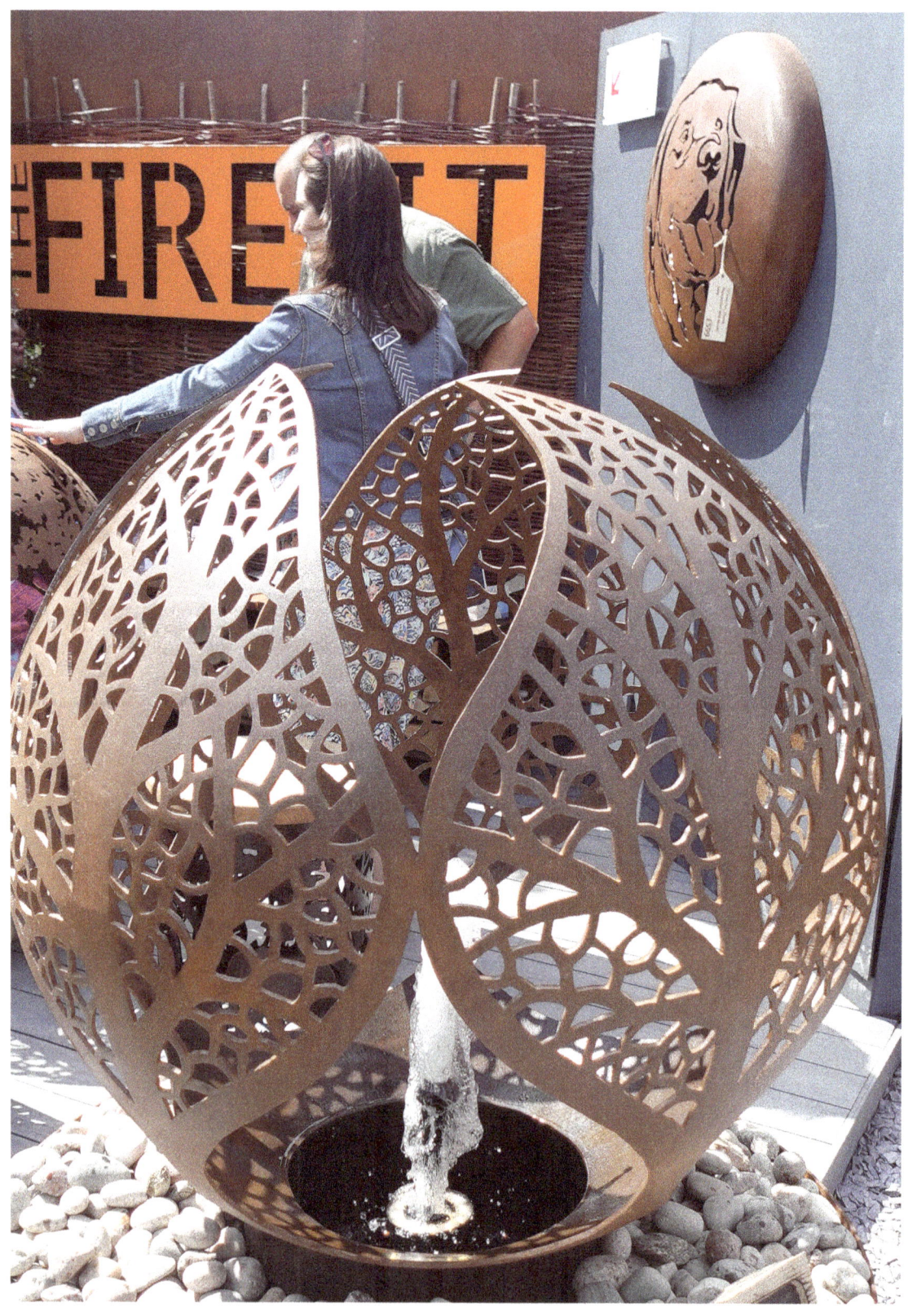

Gentle Thoughts of Childhood

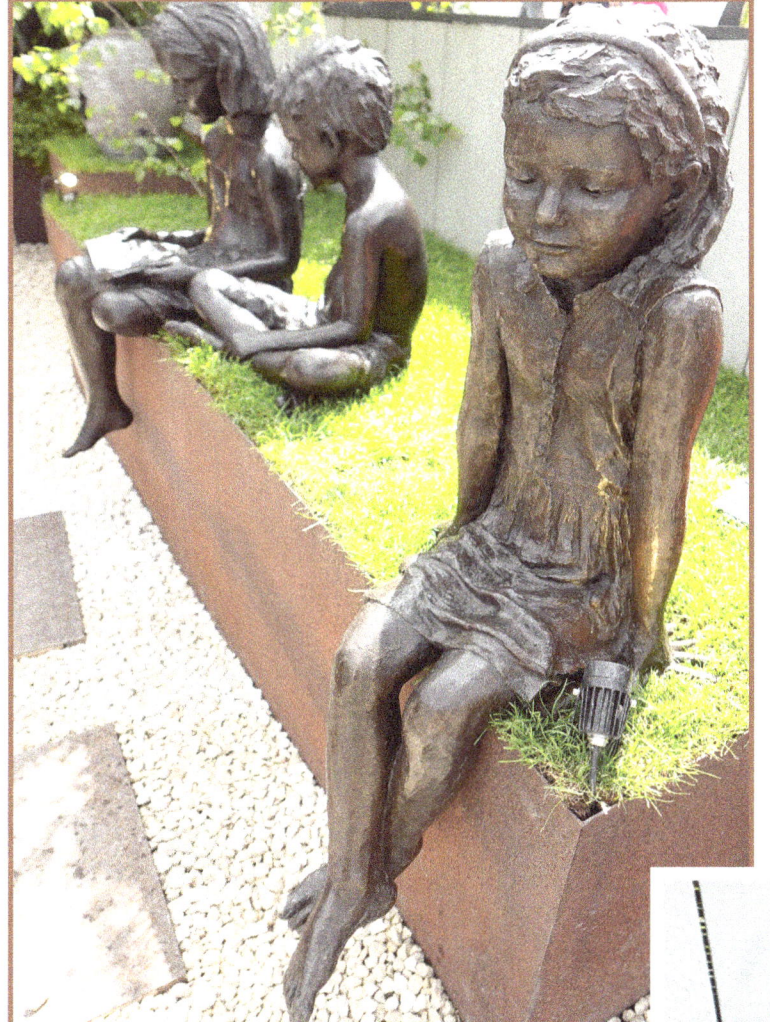

How many times can we reflect on those special moments when we were children?

The peace and solitude of the moment may have been after playing or just taking time to think on a sleepy summer afternoon...!

In these photographs, perhaps, the children have just had a paddle in a cool mountain stream, or maybe, it was just time to take their shoes off after school...!

Whatever the occasion, the sculptures of Brian Alabaster, makes me stop to think of my own English childhood and those very special days of warm sunshine, cool grass to sit on and the gentle blowing of a summer breeze...!

Goodness, what treasured memories these children's images brings to the surface of my mind...!

Hot summer days and the freedom of the countryside all come into the mind as we stop and look at wonderful, and lifelike sculptures.

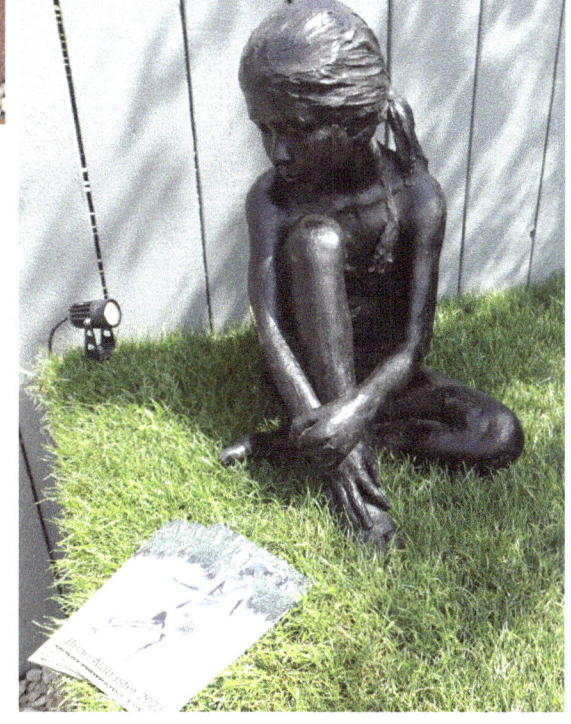

The sculptures show the movement of the children and the freedom they are feeling from sitting quietly reading a book, feeling the pleasure of cool fresh water running on the young and growing body, or from running in the fields; all such movement is seen in the figures we see in these photographs.

The images bring back such bold and vivid memories of an English summer.

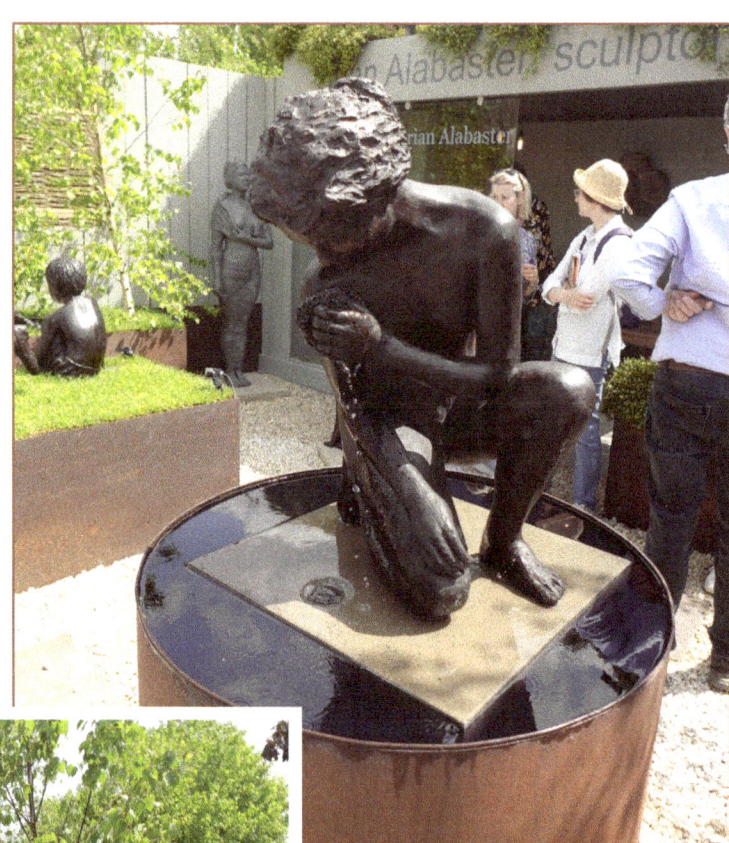

In the sculpture opposite, I can remember my own experiences, and too, recall, my own hair in a ponytail bouncing, as I ran to catch either the bus or running through a field on the way home from school…!

Last year we featured Brian's beautiful sculpture of three children climbing the book staircase entitled: 'The Next Step', this sculpture is now installed in Alperton, Brent. That sculpture was one of the impressions of great physical movement by the children as the climbed each separate pile of books.

A Time to Think and Take a Moment...

Time does not stand still, for the moments of those summer days,
are distant to recall...!

It takes the magic of the moment, and a chance of reflection to
know the journey from that time...!

We may have many mountains set in front of us, and some of us do fall...!

But it is about the moment and the way that we recall...
for many mountains are a hurdle but meant to overcome...!

For that is part of life and sent to make us strong, and yet,
it is easy to find another route...

That was not the intention, and a lesson will not be learnt,
some people feel the anger and some, their heart is burnt...!

It is the lesson of the journey, that makes it all worthwhile, and knowing
if you see it through, many wrongs can be the start of something new...!

For it is in the moment that we hear the magic of the song...!

Do not give up the moment, when life is such a hurdle to restore, but
know that with every moment, there is magic in achievement and helps
you build your core...

Life has many bounties, and some may not know...
but it is the moment and the time to think it through...!

That allows us to be creative in all the thoughts and actions that we take
and do...!

For the magic of the moment, if not understood, may become too few...!

Live, Laugh and Love the Moments.

The Inspiration of Shape

Since the human mind started to collect information and put ideas together, we have been transfixed about shape. Whether it is the shape of the female form, the leaves on a tree, birds in the sky, shape is all around us – shape is shape and has form, is three-dimensional and above all else, incredibly interesting to observe.

These sculptures by John O'Connor, give the human eye a different perspective on the human anatomy.

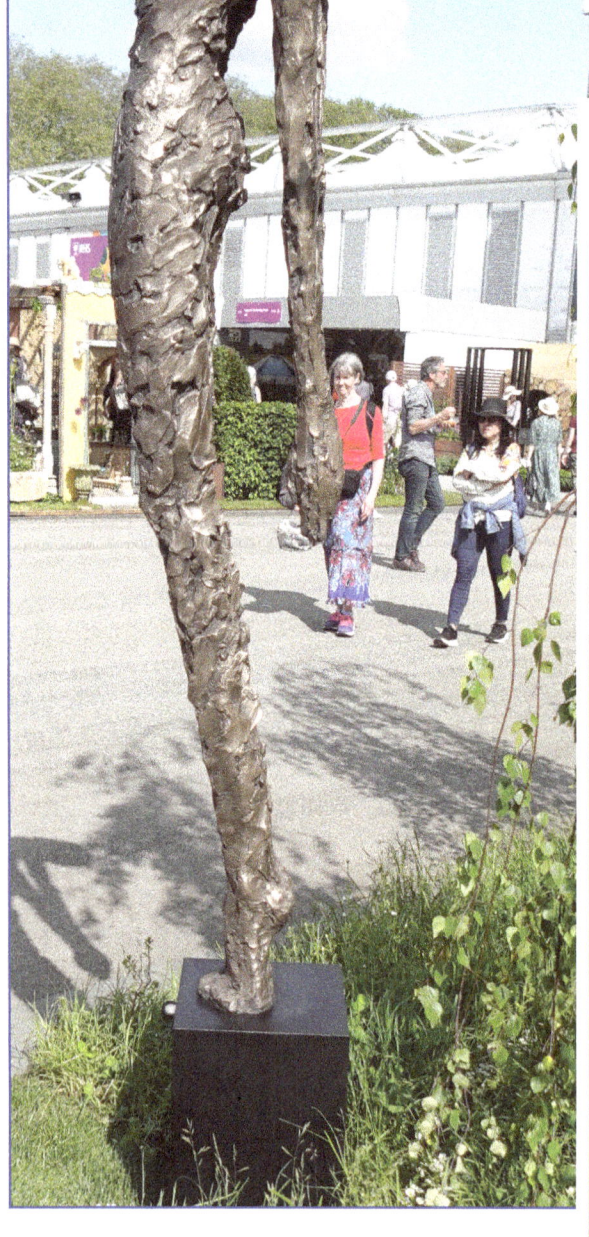

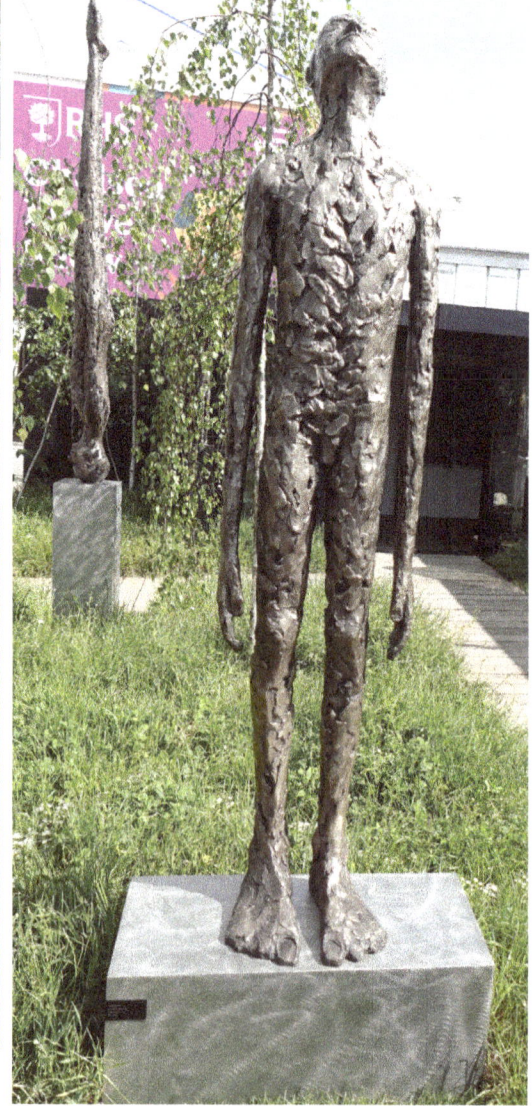

Opposite, is it any wonder we often hear people say, *'I could do that standing on my head...!'*

Regardless of the expression, it is highly unlikely that many people could create such a piece of beautiful art, especially on their head!

In this piece, 'Earth Elevation', the sheer expression within the art form gives us the impression, 'If we think about an idea long enough, we can reach great feats within the human mind and the accomplishments we can achieve.

Opposite, 'Mixed Media' is the title of this sculpture. John uses a combination recycled plastic bottles and highly versatile resin. By adding large quantities of ground dusts to the resins, it offers a variety of finishes.

Some sculptures are produced from iron, bronze, marble, copper, and have slate finishes.

There is a great drive of energy in all John's work. Some of which gives the viewer a feeling of taking off.

Other sculpted pieces lead the eye to the stars, the feelings of magnitude and the wonders we have within our planet of earth. Each of the sculptures lead the mind to thinking deeply about how fortunately we are to be living and experiencing great forms of art.

With such exceptional craftmanship and the insight to create the human form, which takes our vision of the work to extensions of thinking within each viewing, it is difficult to comprehend how a single person can visualise the work and then create it, thus, allowing us all to appreciate the beauty it offers.

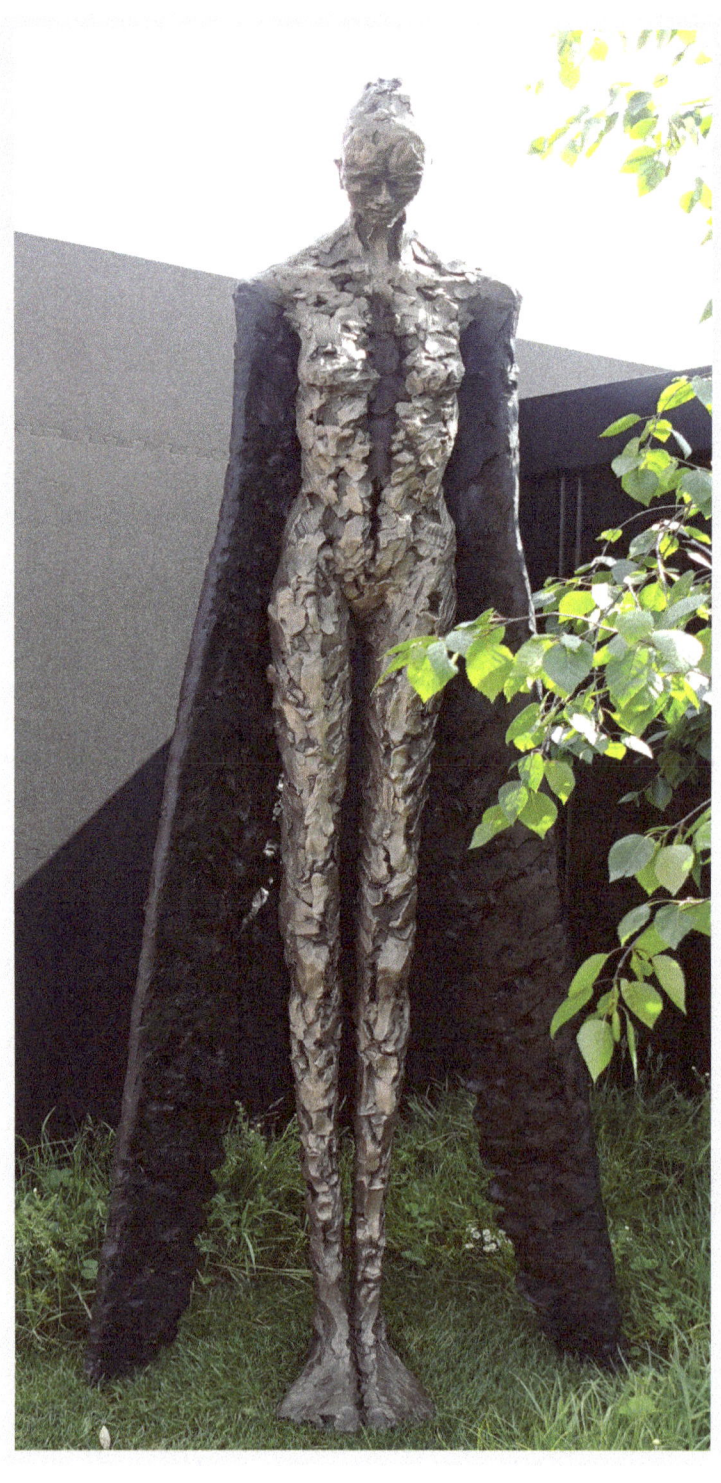

From Flowing Form to the Movement of Glass – A Combination of Glass and Steel

Two such amazing materials working together: stainless steel and glass…!

From time immemorial, the human brain has been intrigued by shape and the extension of how objects are seen and then transcended into images seen on cave walls, or later. Then human capability progressed to cut glass which allowed them to make stained glass windows and further expressions within human emotion.

Every piece of art created, is an extension of the artist's emotion and their perspective of their life experiences…!

Molten glass, when produced, takes a creative mind and many years of working with the medium to understand how glass flows. It is not only the flow but the clever use of colour in swirls that make the opposite sculpture so interesting to observe.

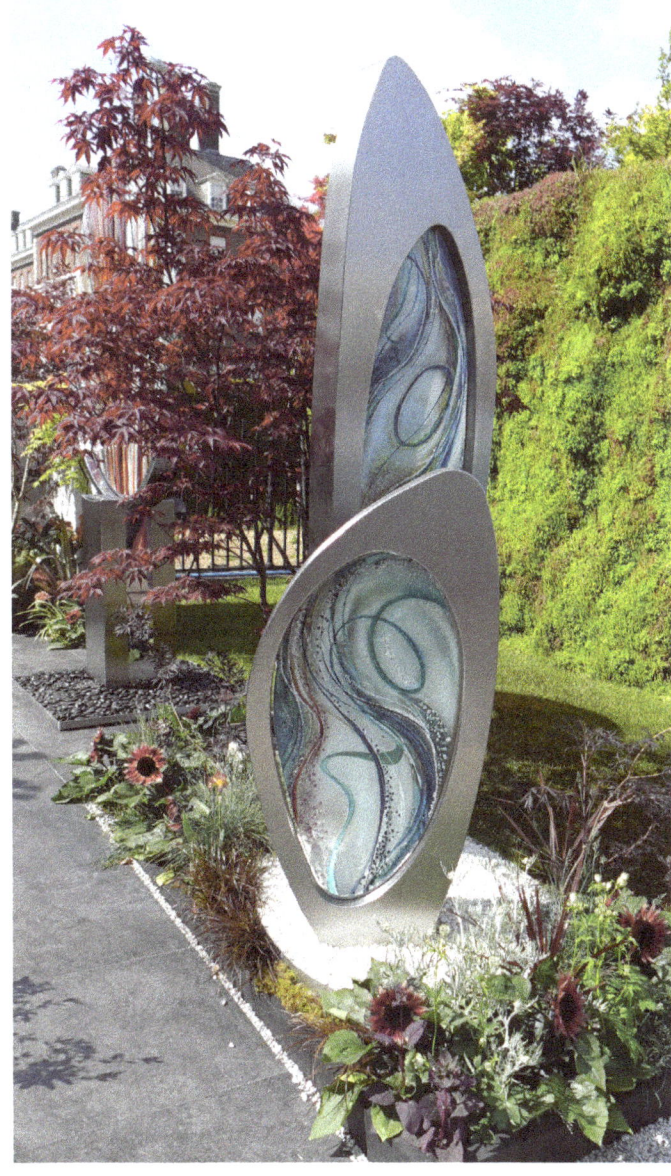

It is as if we are taken back to the running of water, the flow of sea currents, and the mesmerising actions of sea surf, all of which are encased in pure stainless steel. The steel is sharp, definite in shape and almost clinical which adds to the entrancement hidden in the combination of materials used and cleverness in the use of shape.

In the below glass circles, unlike the previously spoken about glass sculpture, that had movement in the swirls and shapes seen, however, this artwork has lines of straight glass seen, all of which are encased in the roundness of a circle. It is almost a combination of contradictions which make the design so interesting.

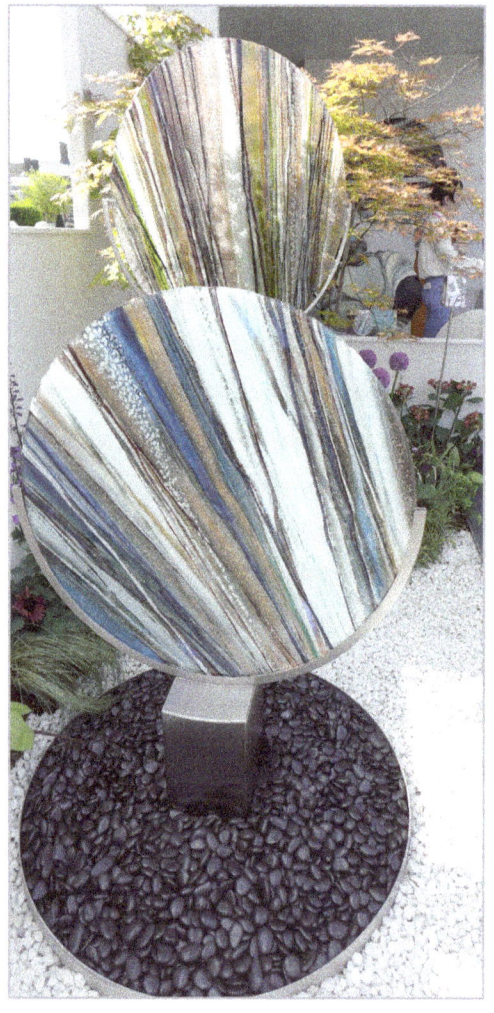

Making a further study of the two circles, one is drawn to the autumn colours of a further round shape, and then to the blues and slight autumn tones of the lower circle.

Introducing blues allows the circle to appear soothing to the eye and yet, the strength of the glass lines draws us to look at the autumn browns which lead the eye to the top circle. It is a clever use of colour when one takes the time to linger and enjoy the energy, work and talent involved in creating such a combination of colour and line.

While at the Canberra School of Art, and during my floristry training, I learnt, '...*a curve is a deviation of a line,*' and in the above the circle emphasises that very description.

Opposite, running water and round shapes of glass are a clever combination used in this sculpture.

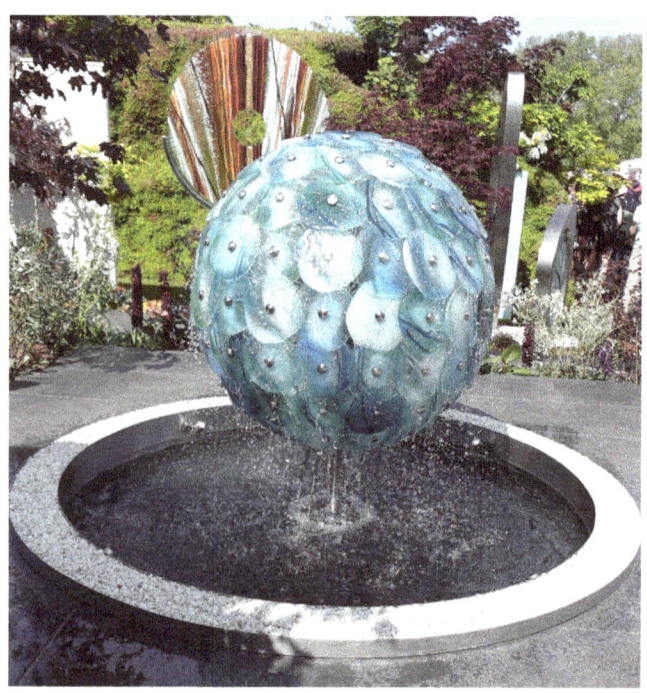

The sound of flowing water can contribute to the wellbeing of our senses: relaxation, peacefulness, and quality brain time...

With Impression – The Merging of Water and Sculpture

As seen in the last photograph of glass, when used as a key feature with water, the combination makes for solace and peace of the human mind.

In the opposite photograph, it is the combination of the water lily shape and the use of water that enhances the richness of the design.

Ian Gill, is both a blacksmith and artist. His work is creative and yet, he can take minimal material to create a combination of movement and expression.

By using creative expression, Ian enhances his ideas into his work which allows the movement of magic to take place. The anodised metal water lily in the above photograph, gives a mystical energy and takes the eye to the peripheral of the design. Adding the water to grey, almost cloudy atmosphere of the visual expectations here, we have a chance to look at the curving petals as the flower unfurls, thus, allowing the water to flow.

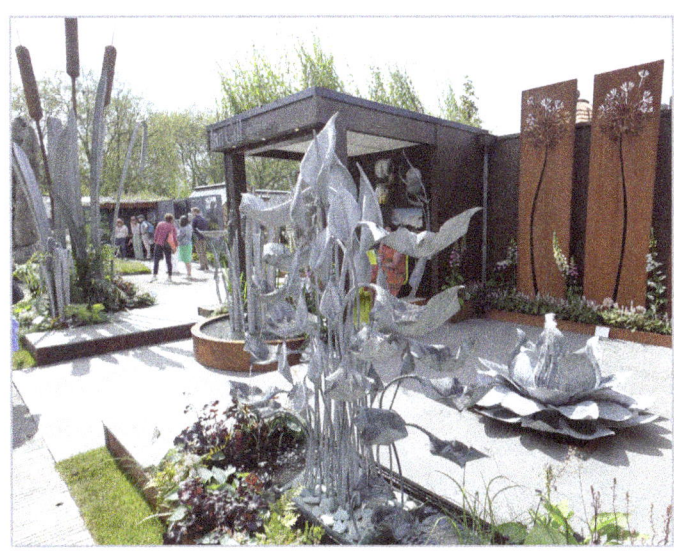

With so many water features in one display, it was difficult to stop looking at the creativity of the moment.

Water, obviously playing a big part in the inspiration and creativity to design and make the sculptures would take many hours of work. Like most art creation, the concept and art form must first be the inspiration of the artist for the design, thus, this would allow creative energy to flow…!

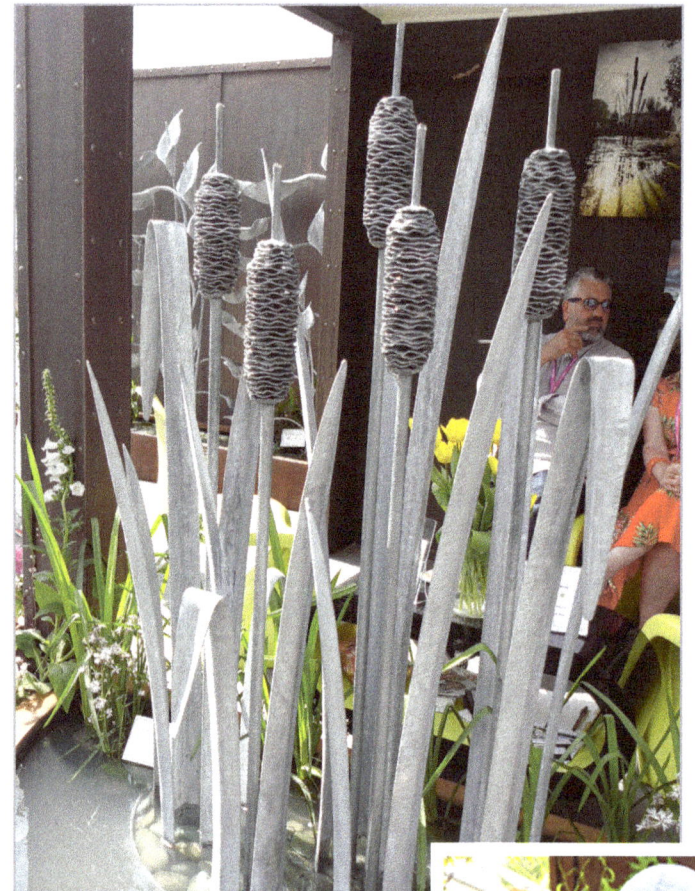

With so much artistic expression from the visual abundance of bull rushes to the image of a nursing mother.

The bull rushes show a combination of water and the significance the water plays of allowing bullrushes to thrive in many natural waterways.

The viewer is led to the movement and humanity of the image below of a mother and child.

The child is an infant; the tilt of the mother's head shows concern and love for the baby she holds.

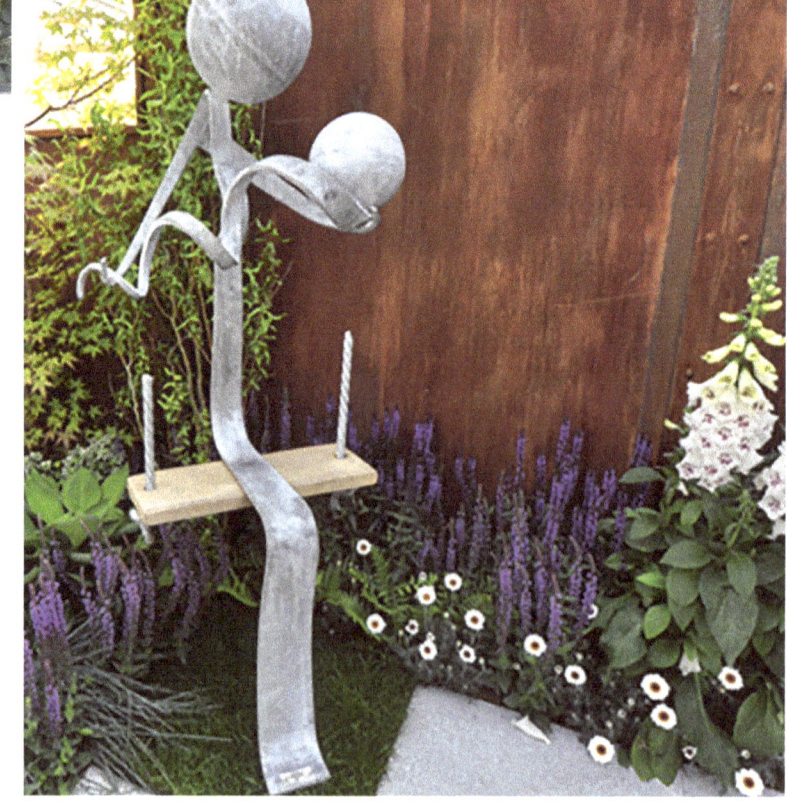

The image is created by using just five pieces of metal, and yet the emotion it evokes in a viewer of the scene is both capturing and memorable.

The fact that the mother appears to be sitting on a swing, in a possible garden setting, also adds to the ambiance of the overall impression one is left with.

From the complexity of natural shapes being taken from nature to the development of the human shape nursing a child can only be seen as a true expression of human emotion.

Paul Richardson

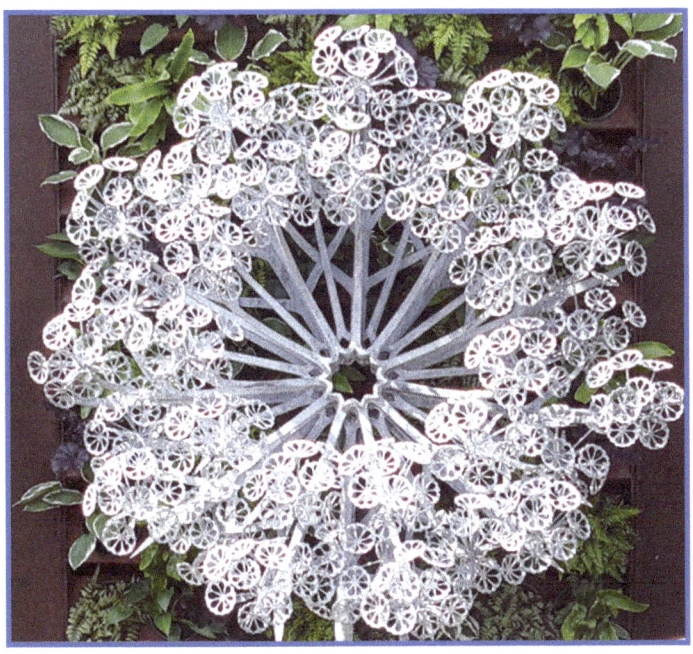

With so much sculpture on offering, it was a bombardment and enjoyment of the visual senses…

Opposite, the zinc coated metal disk shows off an incredible volume of work undertaken to create this almost effervescent image of steel.

With the puffiness of the steel shaped circles, it gives one the impression of a dandelion in seed, which is about to send the seeds into the wind to recreate dandelions for the next season.

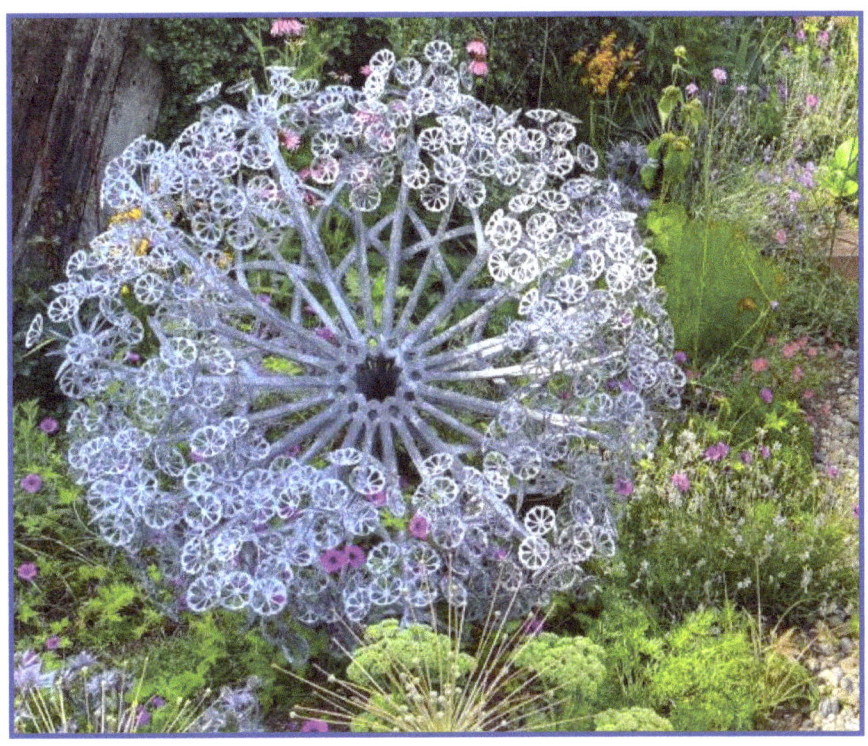

Whilst different light at different times of the day plays an integral part of this delicate design, it should not be forgotten, the sculpture is made from steel.

Photograph courtesy, Paul Richardson, Garden Steel Sculptures

From the Rock it Comes...

The metal it comes from is far from thought...
As we look at the wonder brought...!

When the rock was formed, many millions of years ago...
It was possibly not the intention that art would be created, and there, the human mind would extend and grow...!

And so it is, the creations we have, not only in the artistic light...
but also in the form of war and fight...!

When such beauty can be seen, it is the wonder of the rock,
from which it comes, can be used for inspiration to acknowledge both the splendour and the flight...!

Through past centuries, the rock has been there, without little wonder,
without little care...!

And yet, the human mind extends, with so much emphasis on creative thought, but alas, we can use the rock for both expression and love, and yet, it can be used for none of the above...!

To create from rock, the shapes of unfurling leaves to be seen, and yet, when we stop and think,

That rock now used, can be part of the chain,
and contributes to human pain...!

For without the rock, wars would not exist, weapons would not be made...
and fights may disappear and fade...!

So, the rock we have, has many uses you know, but we should use this raw material for good, so humans can develop and grow...!

Without the rock, the atom would not have been split...
And therefore, the fight that exists between nations goes on,

It is constantly louder than the natural bird song...!

For without the rock, the world would be at peace...

And yet, the digging and extracting of rock, only seems to increase...!

It is the rock you know, that has been given, and yet the human mind is nothing but driven...............!

From Rock...

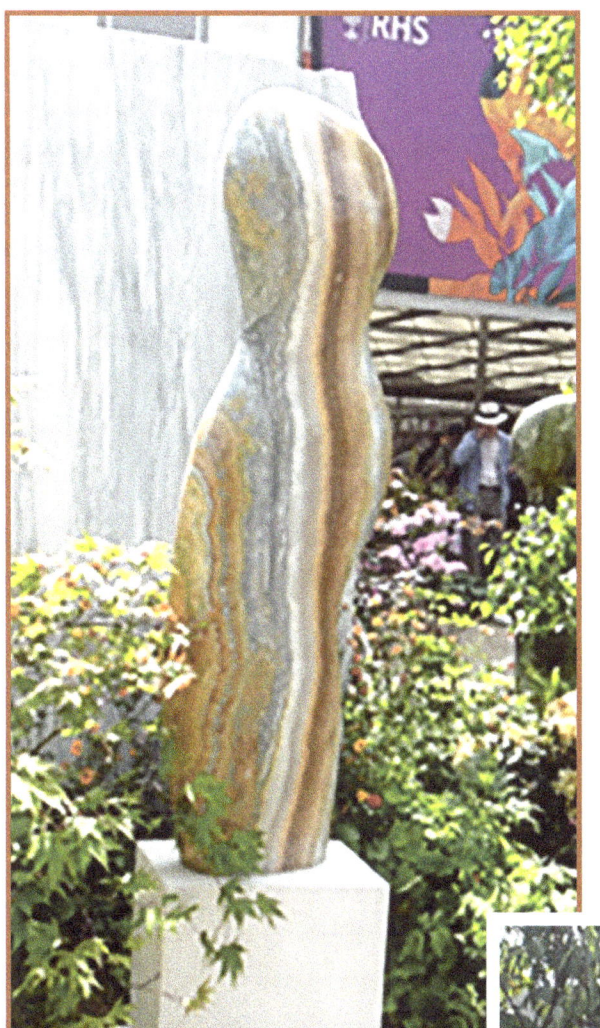

From the shapely female form to other creations from rock! It is not difficult to think of the rock shape opposite as wearing a loose dress by the colours within the natural stone!

Shape, colour and texture bring this sculpture to life and give it movement, dimension and style.

The smoothness of the stone and the hours of work put into creating such a beautiful shape would be many. When one stops and thinks, not one chisel or from a wrongly chipped away piece of rock could be made. The concentration necessary to maintain the regular removal of excess stone would take many hours of work and concentration.

The faces created in the opposite rock formation shows expression and thoughtfulness. To allow the rock the freedom of expression while the shape is created within natural coloured rock formation is breathtaking.

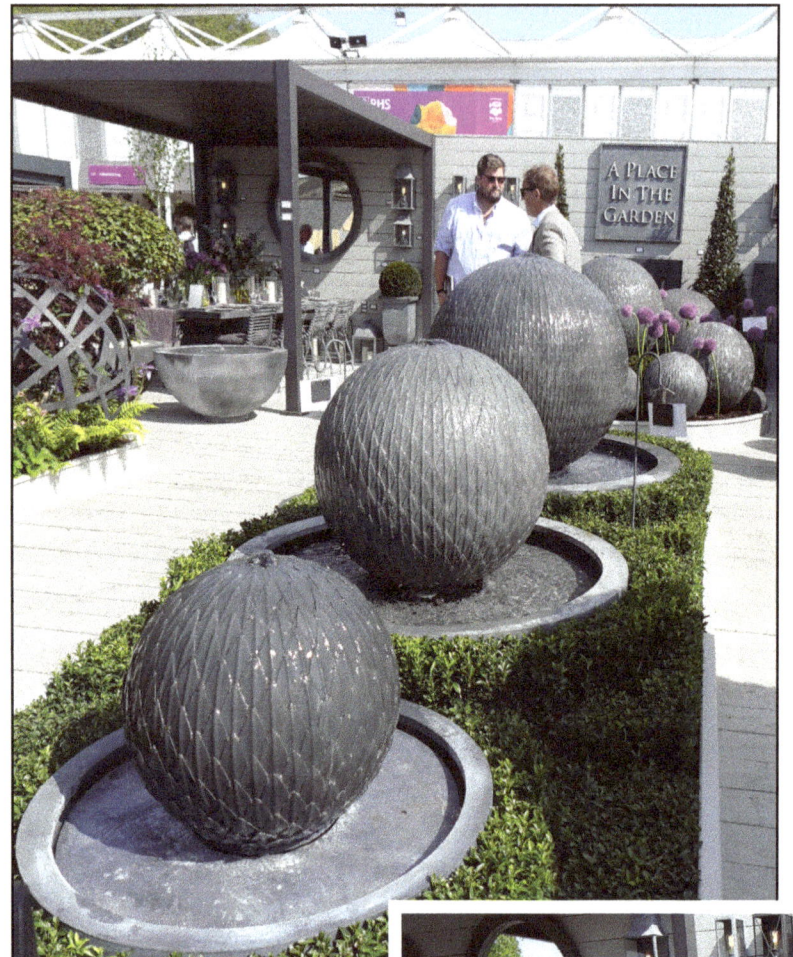

Granite orbs with fine carving and created into water features. The hours of work and carving, chipping away dense rock to form these amazing shapes is almost unbelievable…!

And below, the round grey shapes are complemented by lilac alliums which follow the roundness in shape and form.

The interesting effects of the straight allium stems and the tilting heads of the flowers also add an intererst to the overall display.

The design is clean and fresh with a dramatic play on the colour of the stone, grey and the lilac to lavendar heads of the flower placements.

When one looks deeply into the orbs, we see a whitish hue that shows through the different colours of light-to-dark greys, which have naturally formed over millions of years of naturally occuring rock formations.

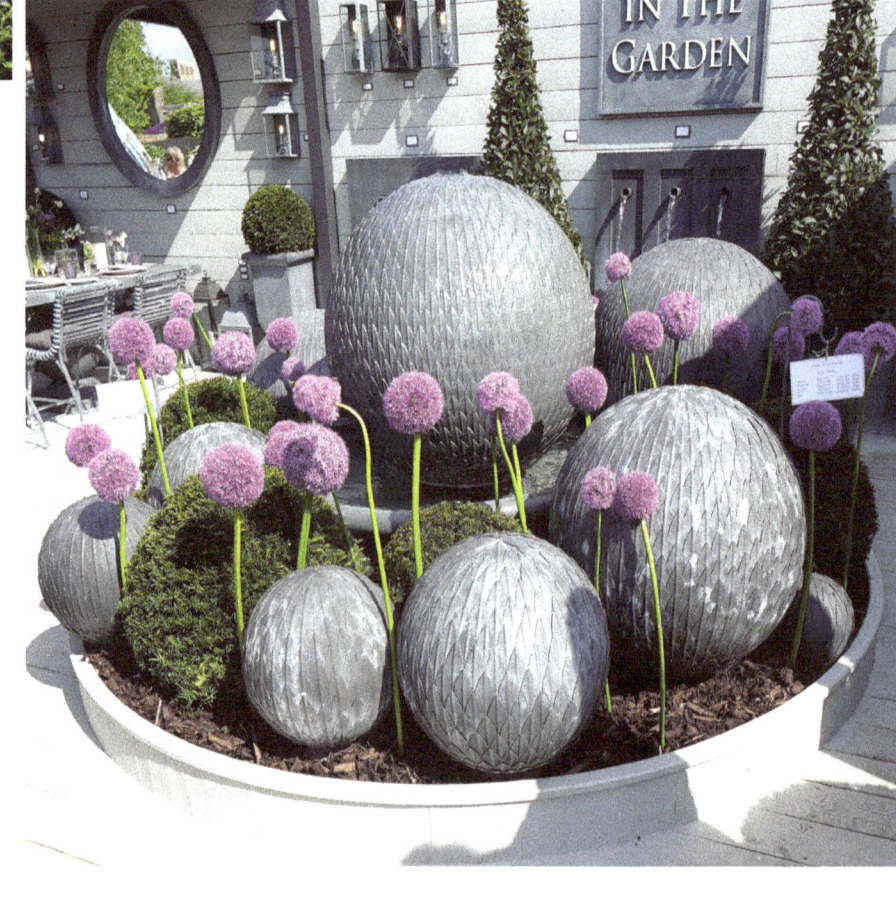

James Parker – Sculpture

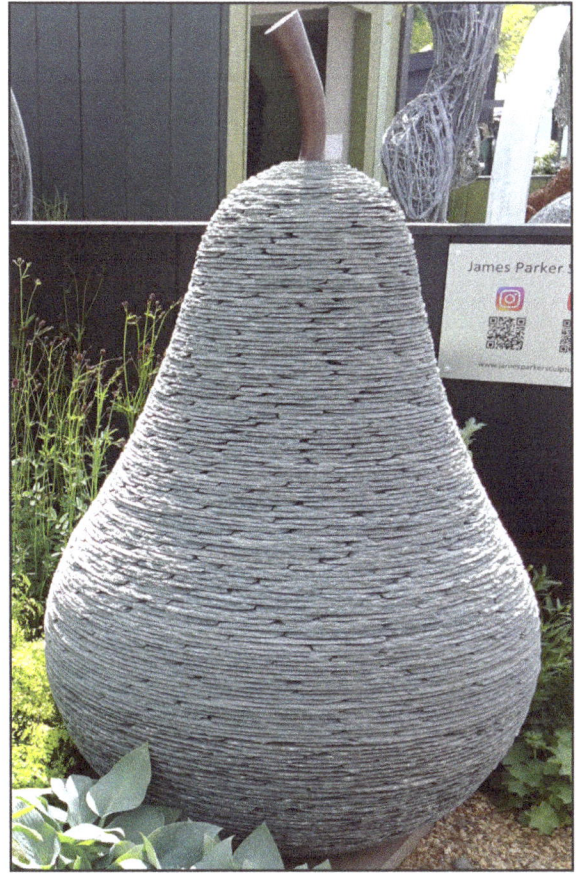

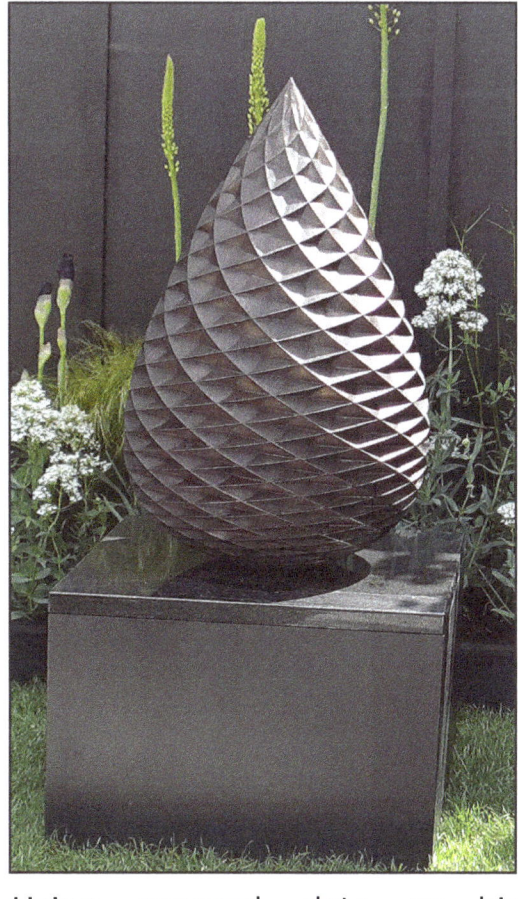

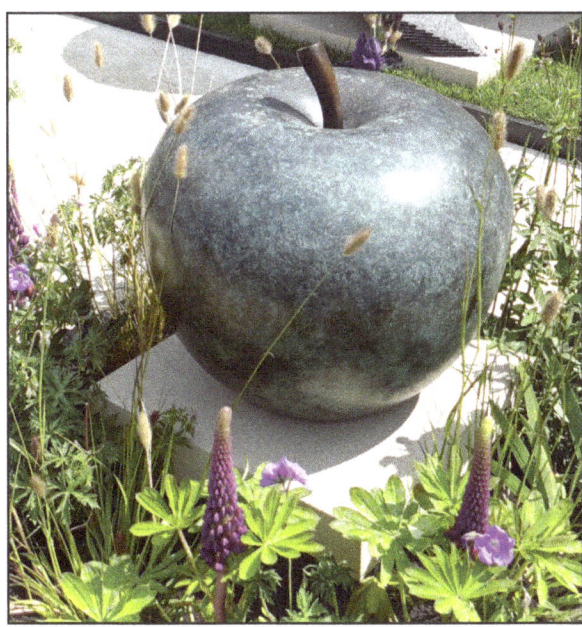

Using exposed slate as his medium in many of the pieces of sculpture, James, creates mesmerising shapes many resembling the fruit we eat and is often found in the fruit bowl at our homes.

James describes slate '...is a wonderfully versatile material to work with. Nature offers an incredible palette with a plethora of colours and textures, from the heather blues to greys, purples, and greens.'

James enjoys using unrefined materials, such as slate, and then his imagination goes to work in the creations he displays.

Slate being a hardy material, it will not let the gardener down. Because of its endurance, many generations will live to see these outstanding art creations.

James continues, 'Form is an important part of my work. Those which are uncomplicated are often the most satisfying; beautiful in their simplicity'.

As James has said, 'slate offers, texture that many materials do not.' As it can be seen in the bottom tiered sculpture, there are many intricate layers, the lower layer supports the next layer and so on. Each layer in its shape plays its own determining role within the design. He further says, 'The layers create depth, the construction is a source of intrigue to many and the slate sculptures I create, rather than dominate, tend to be dignified within, and communicate with their surroundings.'

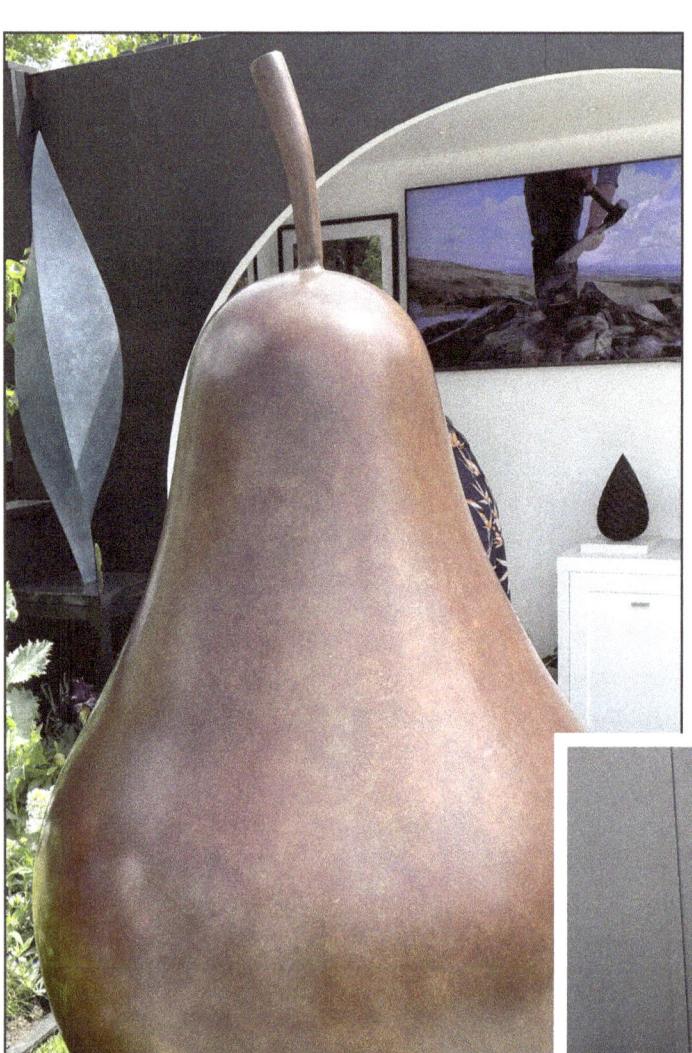

Light in the Garden...

The fascination of having lights within our garden displays brings a lot of satisfaction, regardless of the season!

With so many different shapes and colours created within the garden sculptures, it isn't surprising, we become excited at the possibilities and how to use these masterpieces in our own gardens.

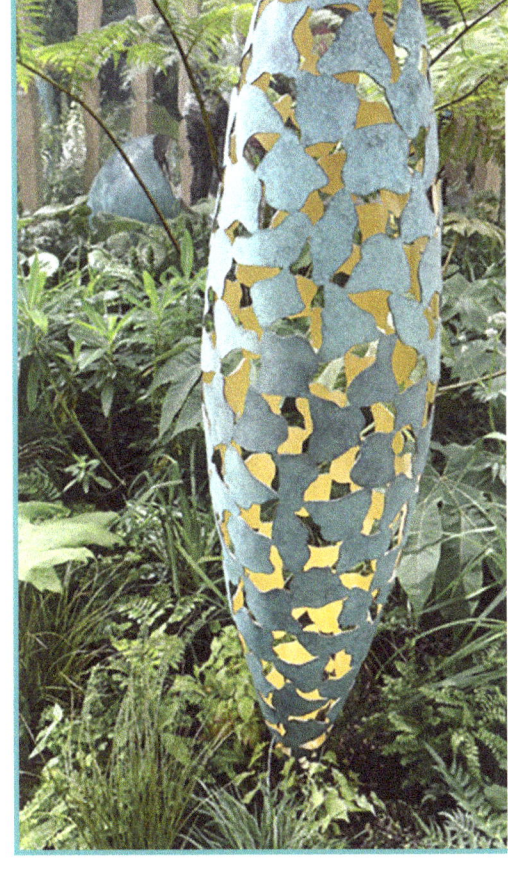

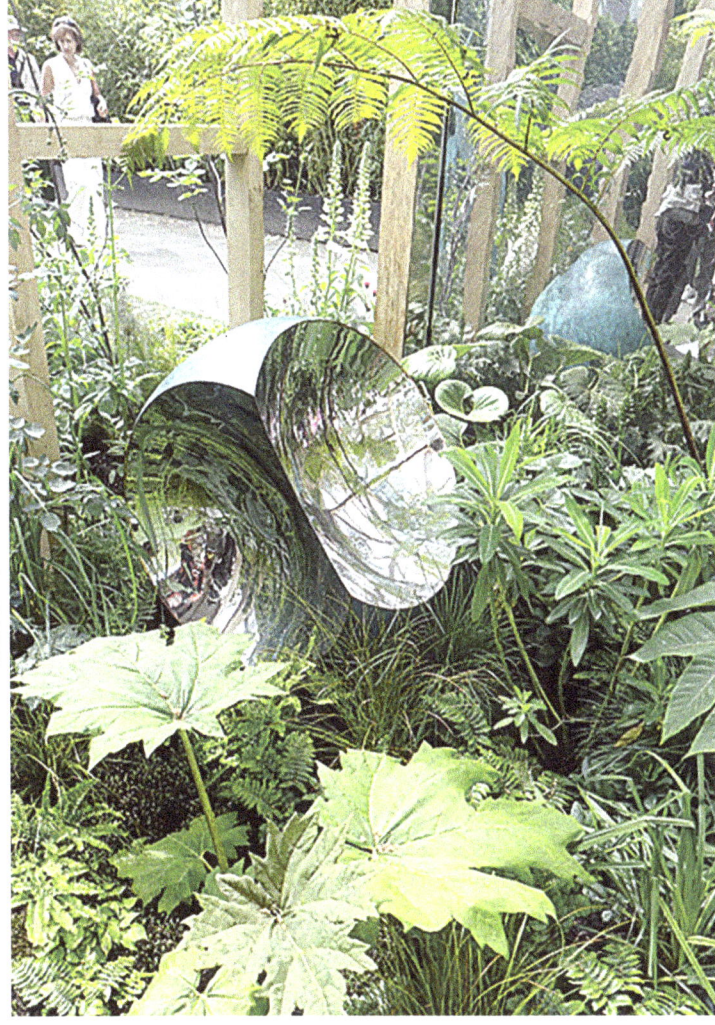

From oblong, pinnacles or round shapes, the garden unique decorations, were at Chelsea, in abundance...!

Reflective spheres, turquoise coloured, round shapes placed discretely within the vegetation of a garden can give an enchanting and mystical atmosphere to any night time setting.

From repeated circles of anodized metal, to long sheaves of repeated metal leaf shapes, all are part of the clever shapes of nature.

By repetition of shape, an artist can make many interesting designs come to life. This repetition allows for interest in visual movement and fascination; it plays with our mind, and we want to look for more, this holds visual attraction, and can be somewhat mezmerising...!

I must admit, I do love sweeping lines in sculpture and design; to me, it adds so much more in form than could otherwise be lost had the shape and movement not been introduced at the time of creating the art form.

A Day of Fun...

A young reporter out to get the best shot of the day! Colour and theme were there with personality plus a warmth that made you want to talk to her; she was a delight to have a conversation with.

It's great to see our young people out on a mission and to achieve their goals.

When asking, 'Can I please take your picture?' Her reply, *'Of course you can!'*

Colour, friendship, and a sense of fun cannot be replaced when attending such an event.

The Art of Floristry Design

It takes many years of study to be a competent floral designer. It is not only the use of the physical materials used in flowers, foliage, and assemblages within each created piece of work, but the clever use of rhythm, space, movement, colour, texture, harmony, size of components, construction, balance and alignment, contrast, proportion, and lastly, emphasis, that allows the florist to become the floral artist they become.

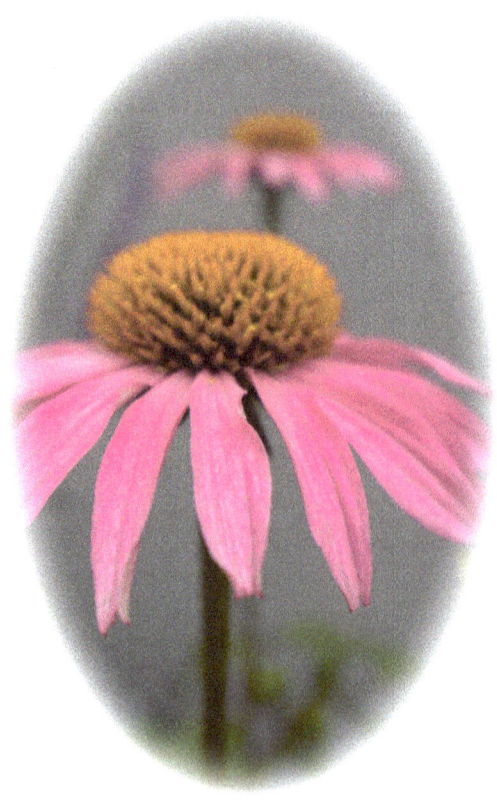

The Art of Floristry Design...

Abundance and celebration are the only categories we can describe the flower designs at this year's show.

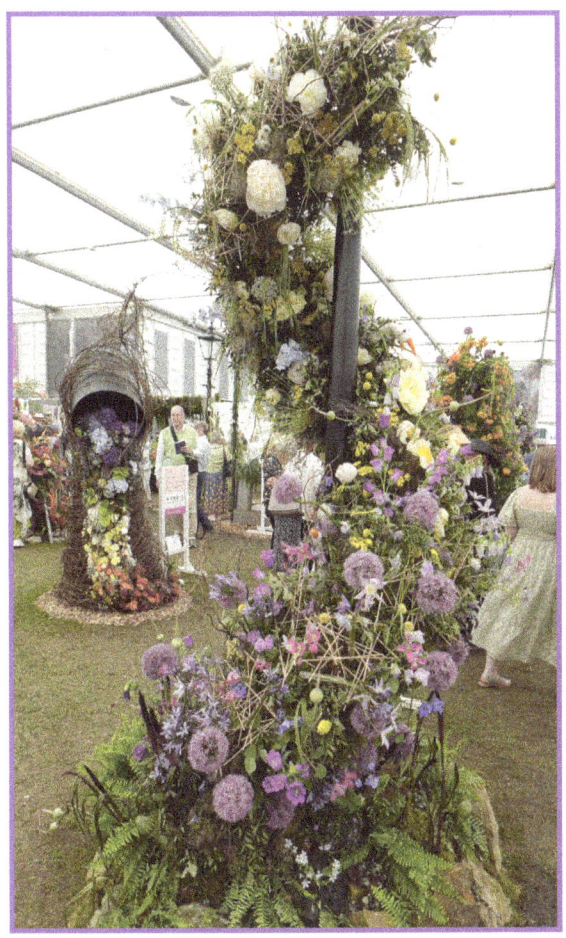

From the Hogarth Curve seen in the opposite photograph using contrasting colours of different tonal values of whites and creams to lavender and purples, with a slight intermission of straw stalks.

To create the Hogarth Curve, one needs to have a firm background in fixed mass floral design and the experience of the artist is seen by the construction and placements within the work. A pleasure and delight to

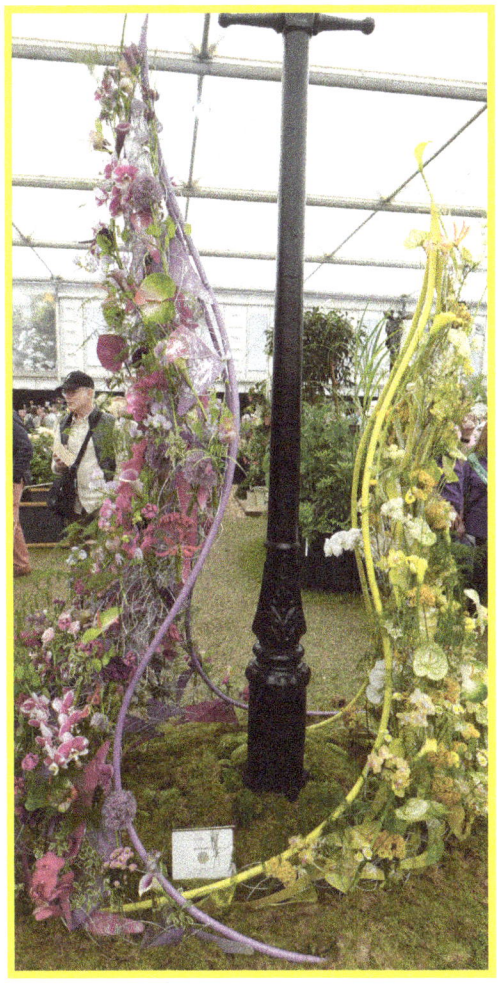

see.
Opposite, the contrasting colours of lemon to yellow and then pinks to lavenders in the two designs opposite is again seen in the Hogarth Curve shapes.

The shapes, not clearly seen in the photograph, are a combination of a pair of reflecting shapes is both visually pleasing and creative.

The unique combination of four designs to form one design, rightfully so, wins a Silver Medal.

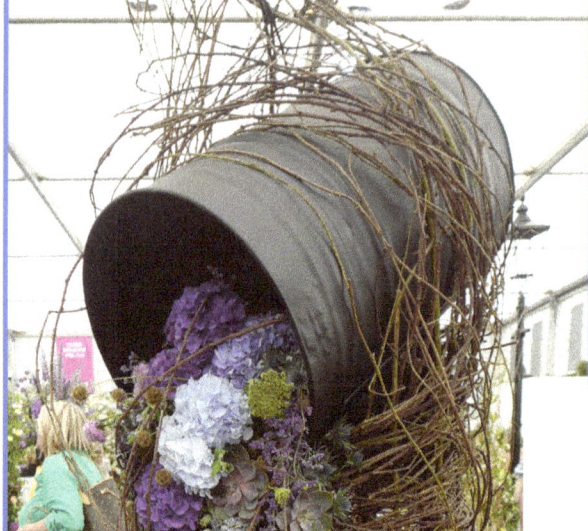

Opposite, with so much emphasis on renewable and recycling, this drum has been put to good use.

The hydrangea is an old-fashioned flower and is greatly appreciated by most floral artists, whether working within the commercial floristry industry, or in the local floral art clubs and organisations.

With colour blocking now seen in many floral designs, it's a relief from the coloured speckling that used to be so popular.

By mass colour-blocking, we not only enhance the floral designs, but add visual impact to each design we create.

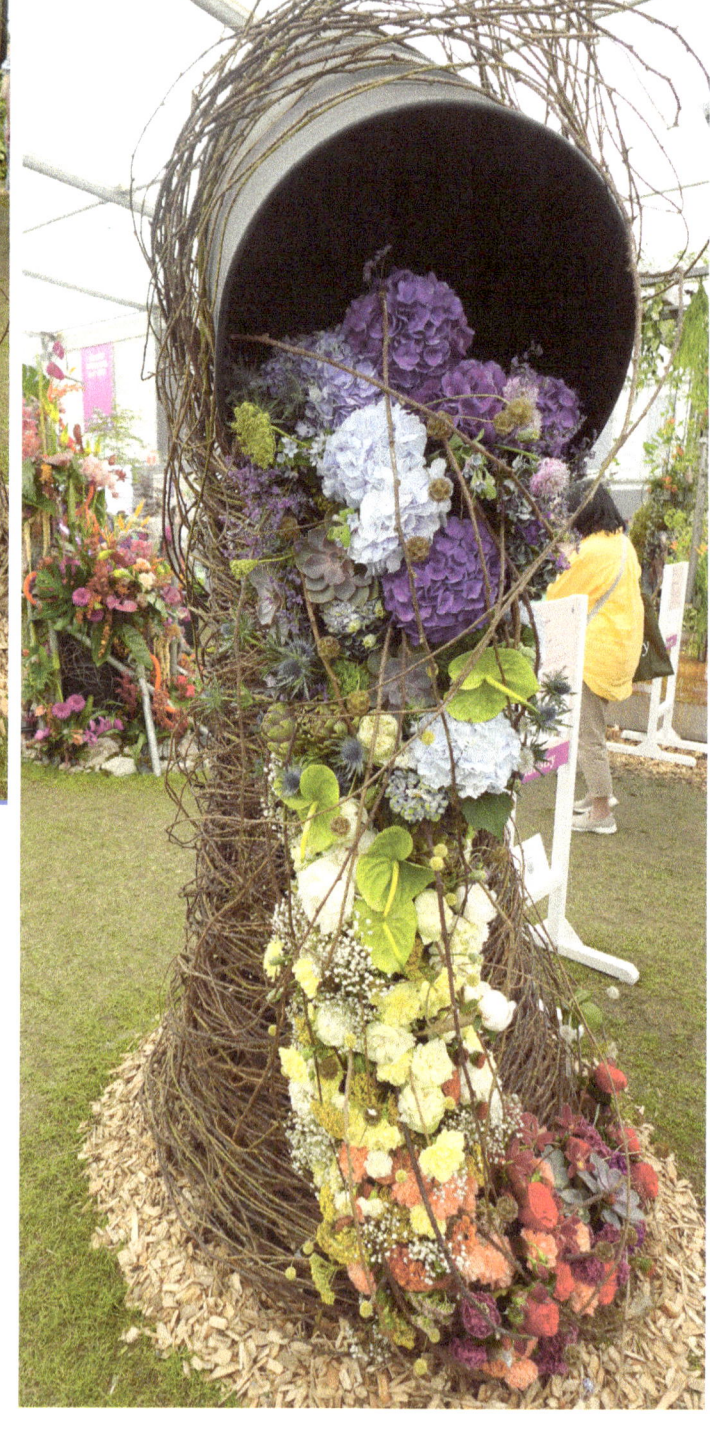

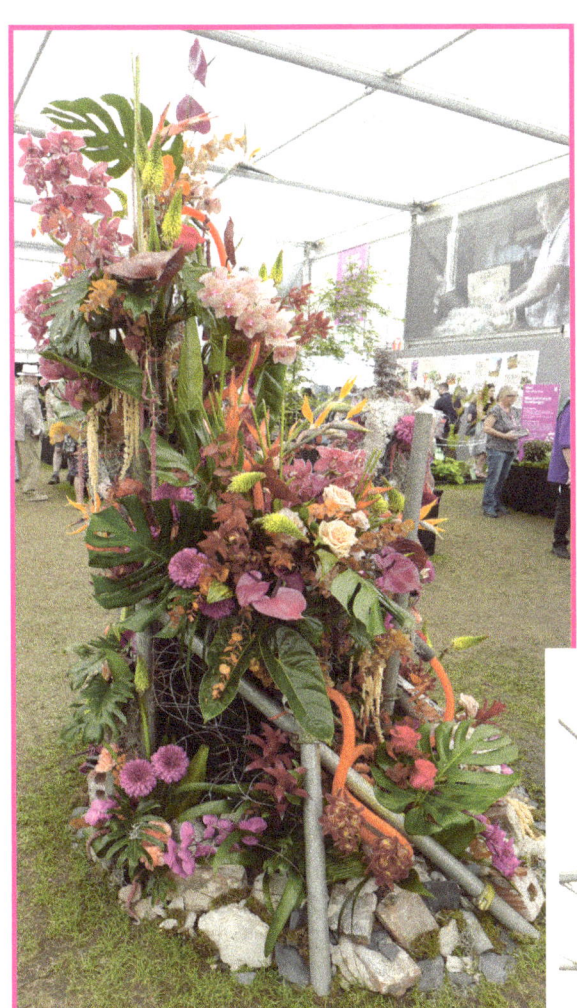

Opposite, the vibrancy of colour and creativity are not readily seen within any photograph. The mass effect of the flowers in oranges, pinks, and reds with gushing Cymbidium orchids from within the design, and then tying the work together is a bendable red tube.

There are many beautiful flowers within the design; at the lower end, towards the base of the arrangement, are purple dendrobium orchids, salmon-

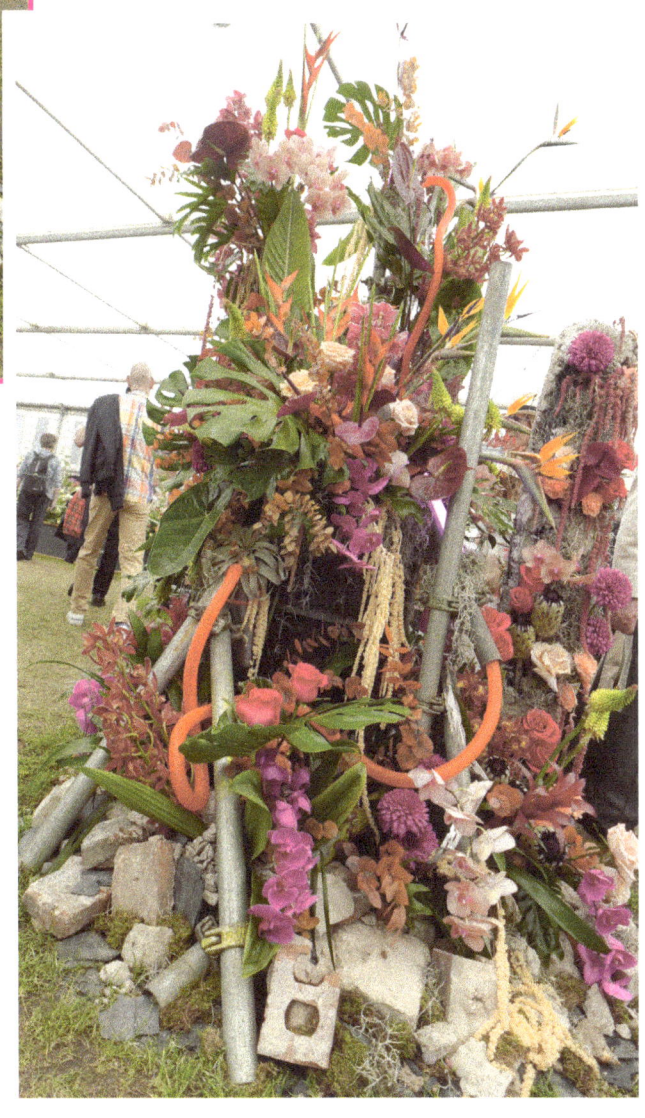

coloured roses, and occasionally seen are strelitzia flowers.

Giving the design an almost semi-industrial appearance, a piece of scaffolding; by adding the scaffolding, the shapes are harsh in appearance when compared to the delicate and almost whimsical appearance of the flowers, and the supporting leaves that, not only break up the flower colour but also the flower shape, texture, and appearance!

The mixing of hard rustic rock also seems to stabilise the overall impact.

Below, the use of colour, texture and movement encapsulate the visual impact of the presentation.

This 'Gold' winning arrangement, titled 'Botanical Spillage' has cascading flowers and foliage making this design sing. The weeping green Amaranthus, striking oranges, purples and lavenders are blended in this mass vertical design giving a sense of mass and abundance.

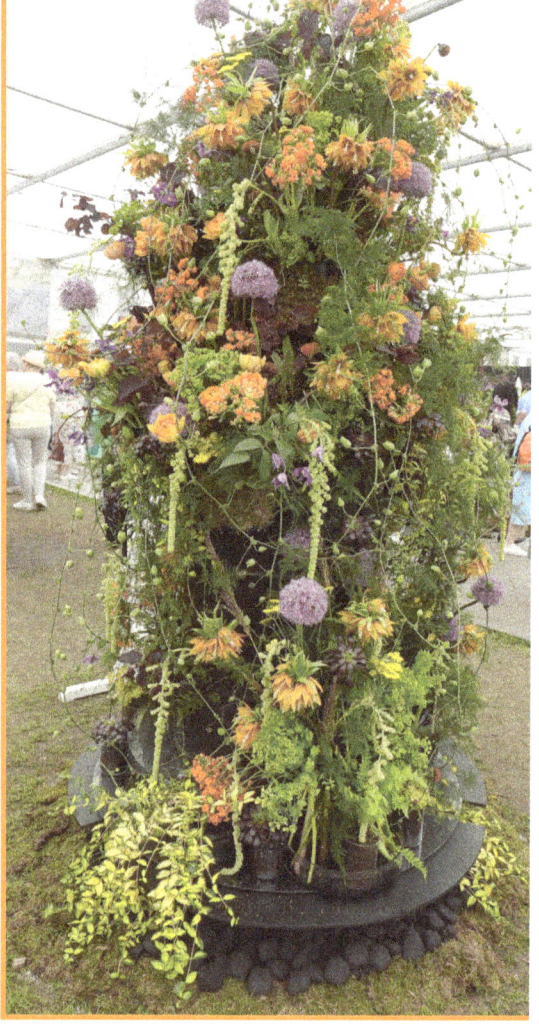

Purple alliums, sweeping tendrils of unopened orchid spikes, and a mass of different coloured orange flowers, including double-parrot tulips, are pushed together to make this splendid mass display. It was nice to see plumosus asparagus fern being used in the 21st Century; it was a fern that lost popularity several years ago; it gives a lightness, airy and ethereal presence to many flower and wedding designs.

Please keep in mind, asparagus may be toxic to cats.

Below, a framework of cane supports this arrangement of mixed and different foliage with a mixture of perfectly placed light field flowers; this blend makes this design delightful and a pleasure to see.

With a combination of different whites, to cream, apricots, and

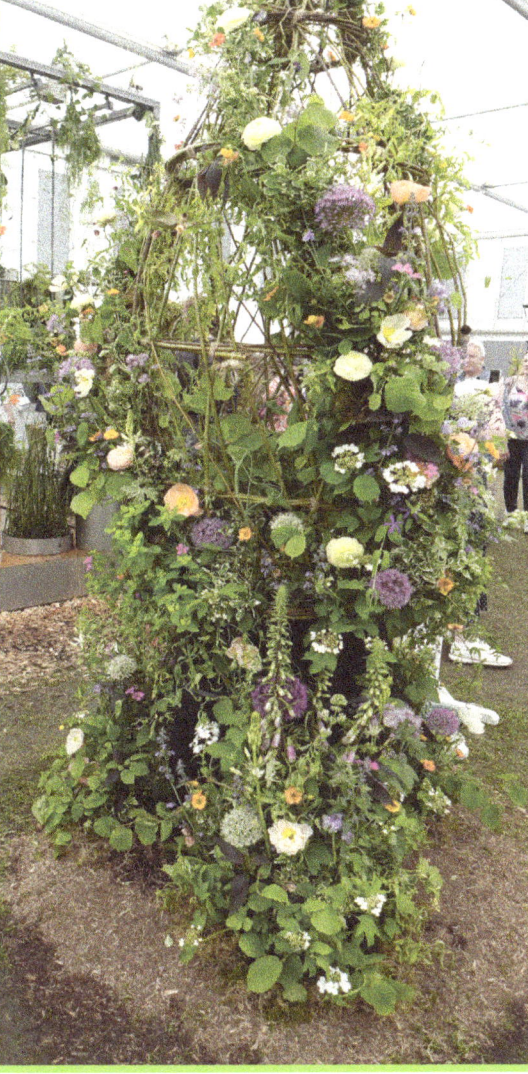

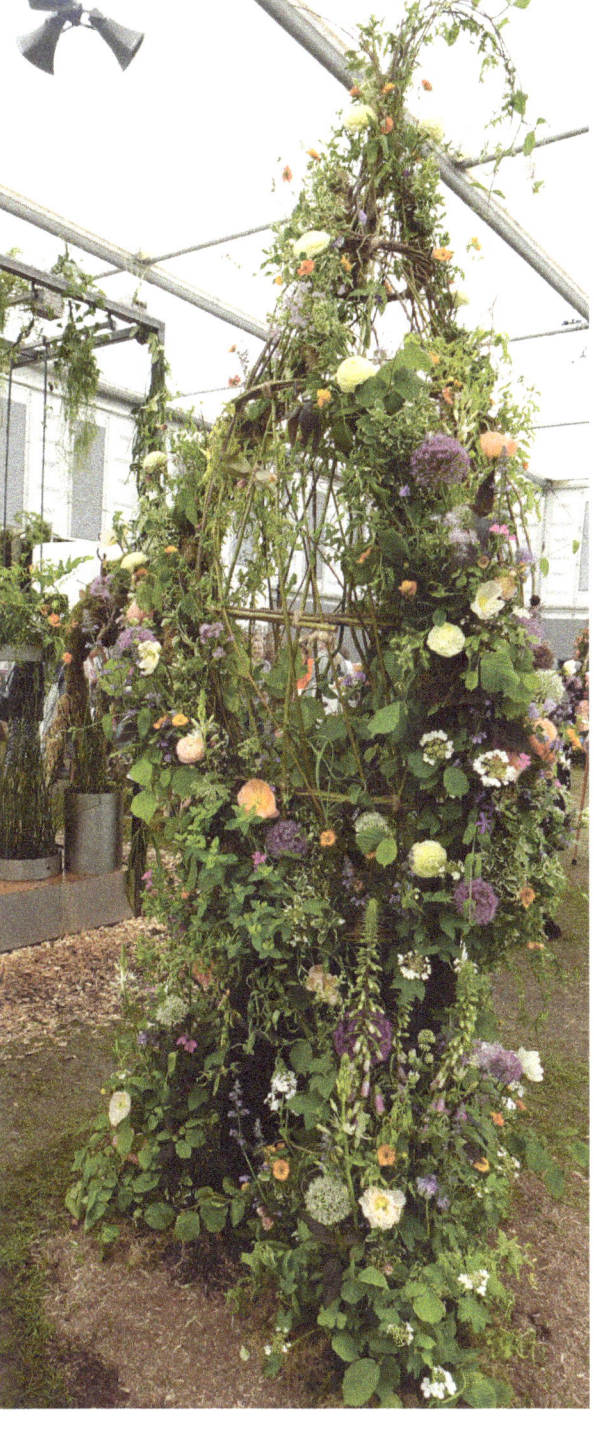

different tonal values within the lavenders to purple hues, and the added textural value of small alliums, all make this a soft and tranquil design that is very pleasing to study and learn from.

The void towards the centre of the design helps to keep the soft and dignified appearance of the completed work.

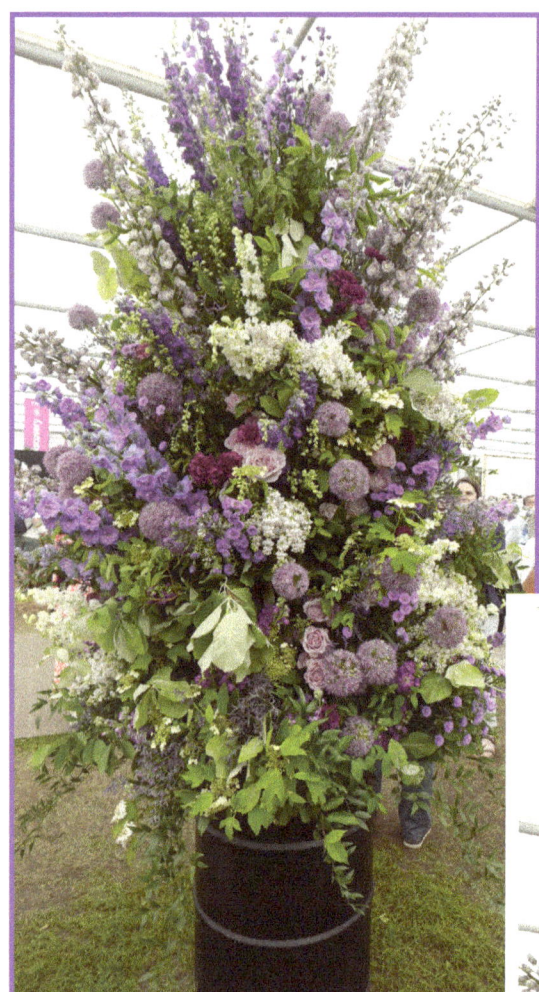

Opposite, the 'magic of the moment' was caught in this amazing, traditional mass design.

Leaving the viewer with the 'Wow...', '...*please show me some more...!*' feeling, it was the essence of the show this year: abundance, but not extravagant or garish, but fun and colour.

From massed delphinium flower heads in soft, and blushing pinks, to larkspur and dusky-pink roses, all used in blocked colouring; blocking adds to the impact of any design whether large or small...

Lavender alliums, white larkspur, purple Easter daisy, and the newness of young summer green foliage all add to a majestic and impacting display in the traditional massed design.

The anchor the work, again, an old metal drum has been repurposed, painted black and used as the container. The design leaves a positive and pleasing impression with the viewer.

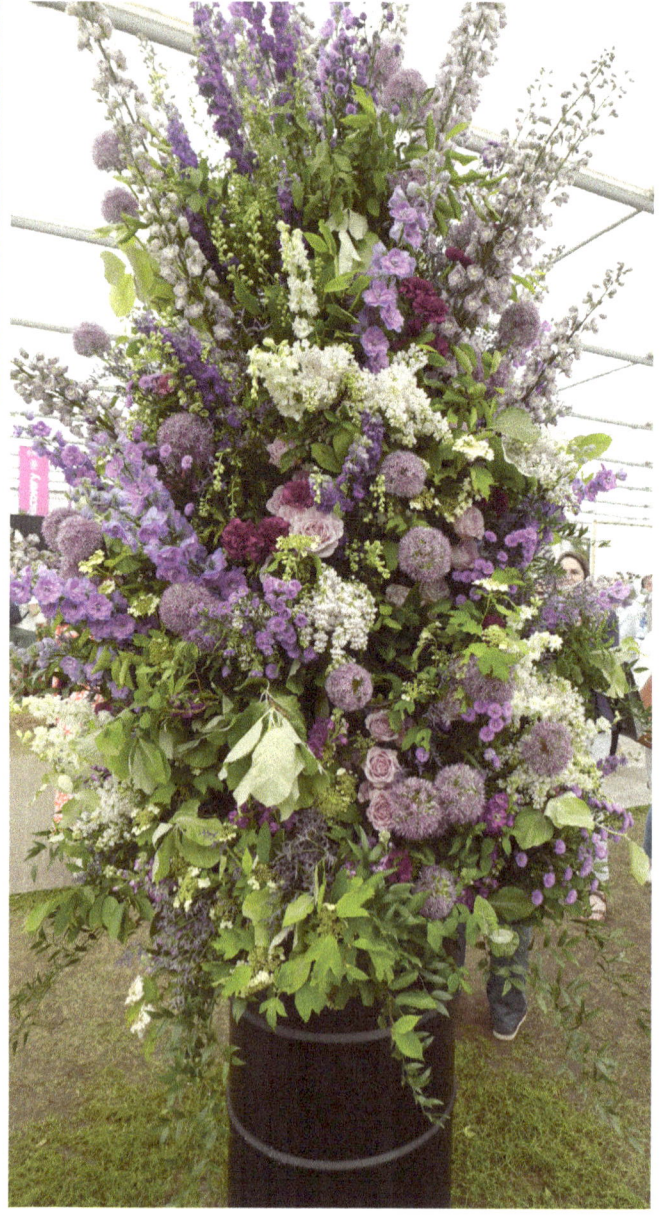

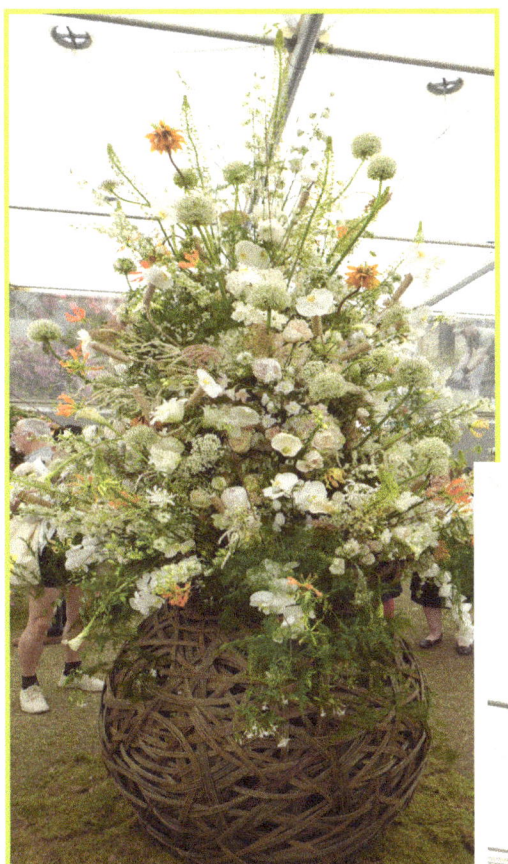

Moving away from the colours of purple and pinks, opposite, it was inspirational to see whites and creams brought together, these colours being interspersed with apricots and oranges.

The anchoring down of the woven basket shaped container, helps to bring about the overall pleasing appearance of the arrangement.

With cascades of flowing white phalaenopsis orchids, white allium, and what appears to be long rolls of natural cotton, white arum lilies and again, plumosus asparagus fern being used.

The sheer abundance of the design is breathtaking and interesting to see. The movement of texture, colour, form, and expression are all about the working components within the design.

Gloriosa lilies also play their part in demanding to be noticed in the vibrancy of the orange colours seen.

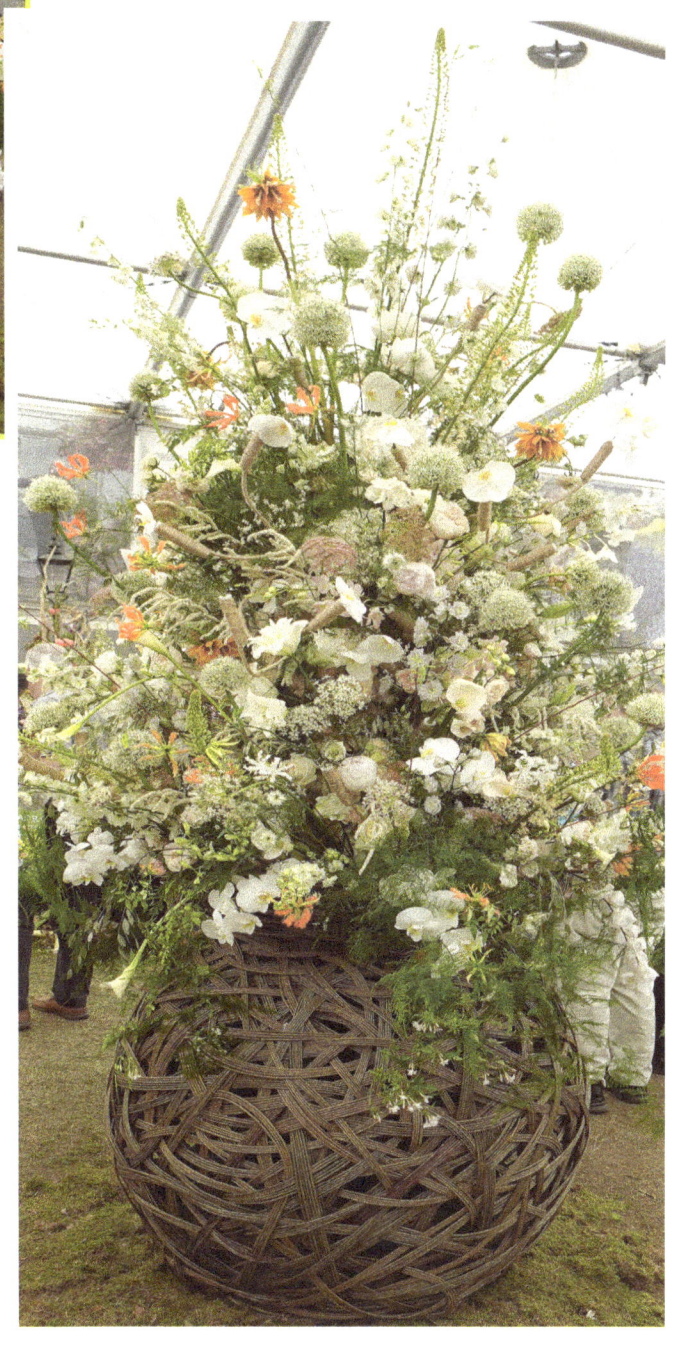

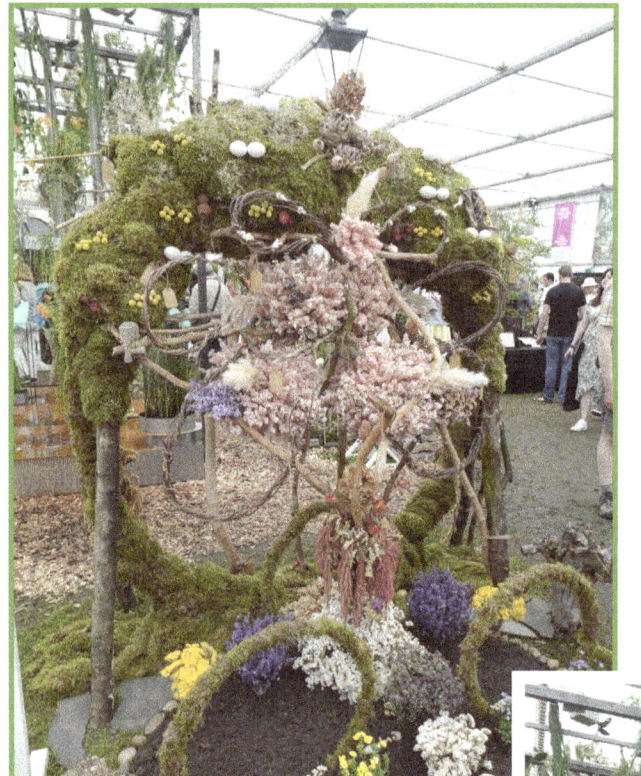

Opposite, a very different approach from the traditional massed flower arrangement was used in this design.

The centre of the design gives the appearance of pink coral and hints of the world's oceans and yet, the abundance of moss with pairs of egg placements, suggests the beginning of new life.

Dashes of yellow also add an interest, while the circles seem to resemble the world going through its different motions.

The rocks to the left edge also play a role in adding different colour and texture to the design.

The eye is drawn to the centre, coral-pink placement, which again could suggest the sea and the start of all life from the very beginning.

This was an interesting and very different approach to interpretive floral design and work.

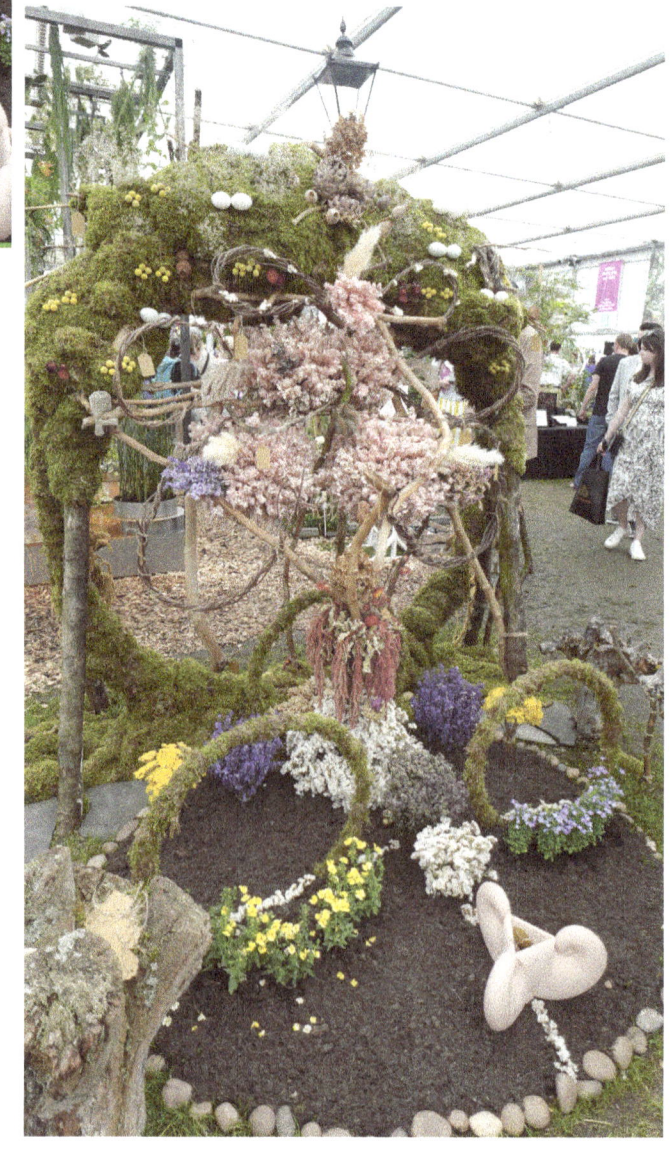

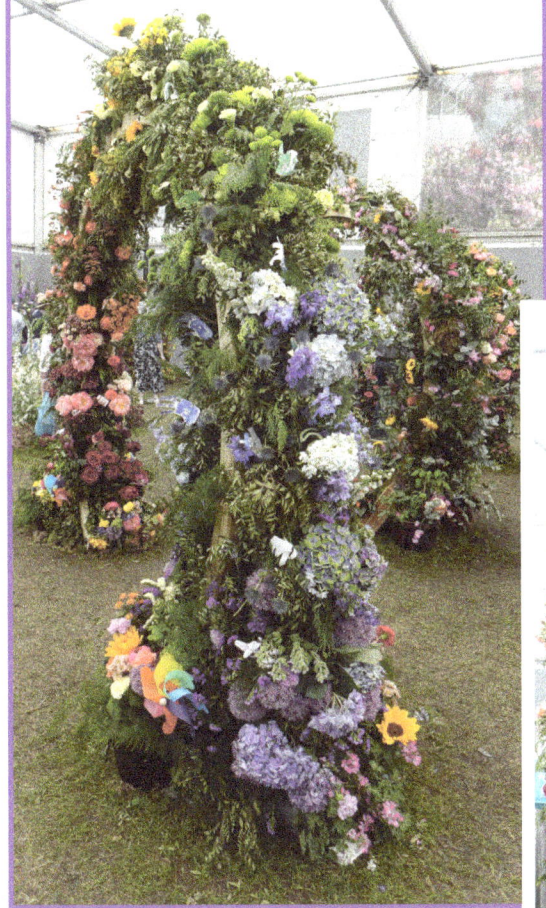

Opposite, the magic of the semi-circle in floristry design. Circles, semi-circles, and the use of curves in any floral arrangement always adds a touch of mysticism to the creation.

Unlike many other mediums used in

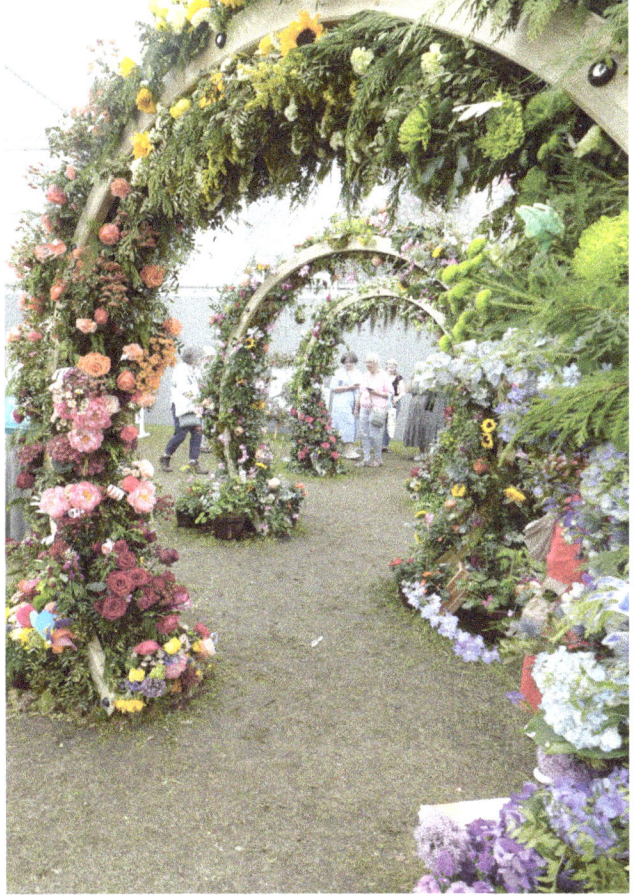

the creative arts such as clay, paint, marble, metals, and other materials, 'flowers are of the moment...' Once their beauty has faded, they are no longer of the moment...!

It is this intangible aspect of flower design and arranging flowers by the floral artist that keeps the floral artist's interest. It is the challenge as they strive for new and different designs to create, and different flowers and foliage to use; their determination to create something beautiful that can never be created a second time, regardless of how the artist will try.

I have tried many times to re-create a floral design and regardless of how hard I have tried; it cannot be done. Something similar will emerge, but it will not be identical!

When looking through the floral archway corridor in the above, one cannot help but think of perhaps, taking off the walking shoes, and skipping through the floral display. An abundance of colour, movement and creativity is used in this spectacular design.

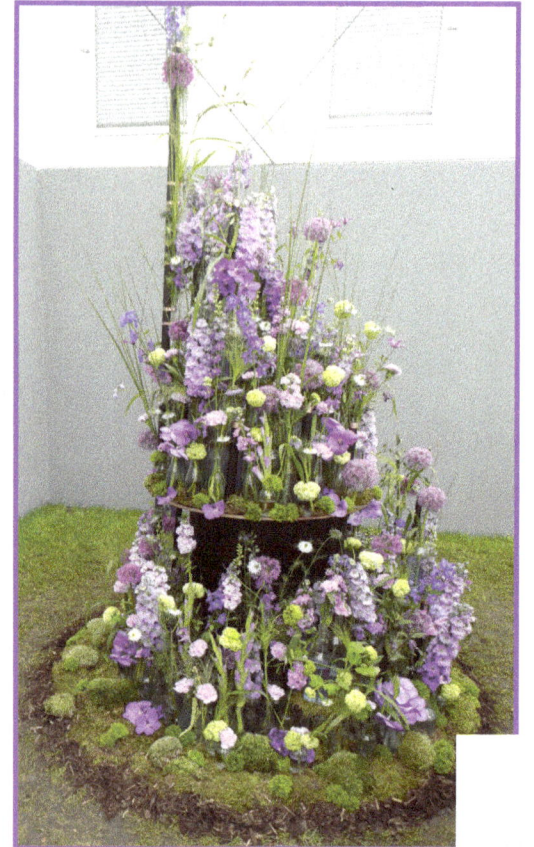

Opposite, and below, is a 'Gold' winning design, titled, 'The Beauty of Recycling,' is of lilacs, lavender and purple, with just a touch of chartreuse; thus, a combination of peace and stillness with using colour! With so many of the cut flowers sitting in singular bottles, the design will remain fresh for many days; this is a new approach to floristry.

With two tiers adding to the mix of the design giving a view of abundance, harmony, and dance. The use of moss adds in the grounding necessary to let the viewers know that the flowers are growing; they are fresh and have life within their form.

We are now seeing recycled bottles and many other recyclable objects being brought into 21st Century floristry, surely, this identifies the concerns of waste products, land and sea fill that are prevalent within our world environment!

Even in a busy flower show, I have found, within these colour combinations, the peace that is given to my brain, through visual satisfaction, is extraordinary.

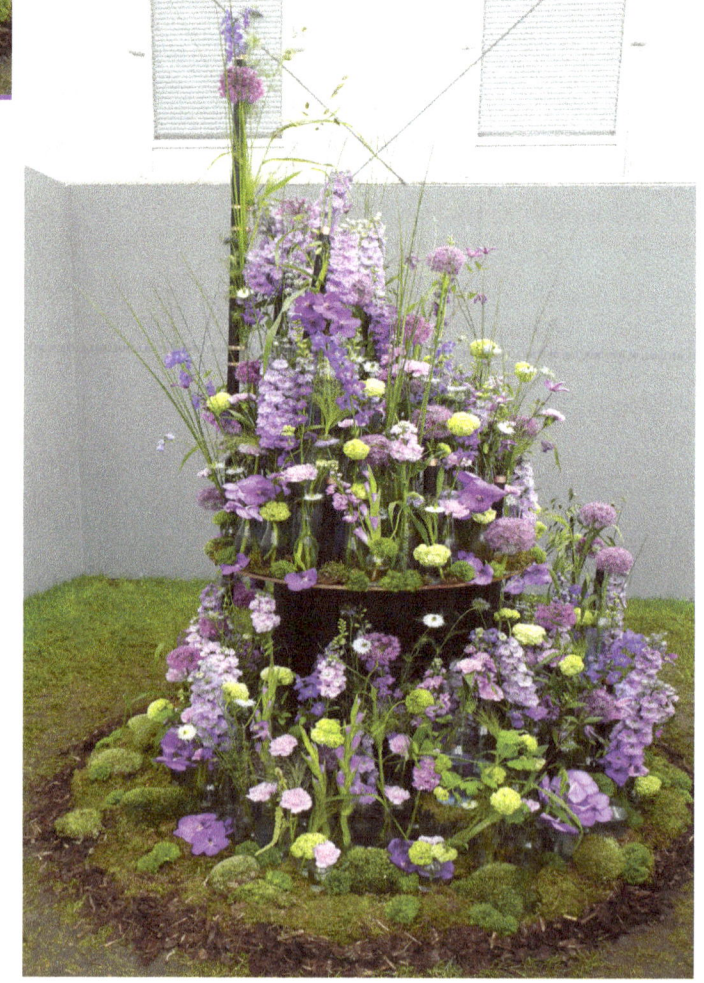

Below is a combination of pleasing satisfaction.

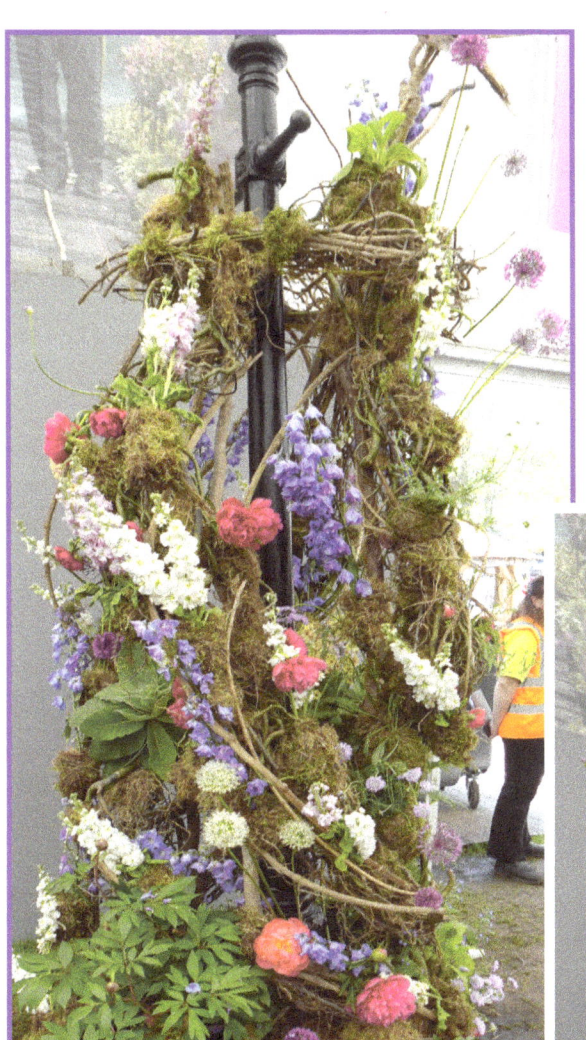

When one takes the time to look, study and identify, there are swirls within the placements of flowers, cane, and foliage. Each placement leans to the left of the design, with the cane leading the visual way through the arrangement.

Vines, moss, and cane are integral to the flow of the design. The solid shape and placement of columns of

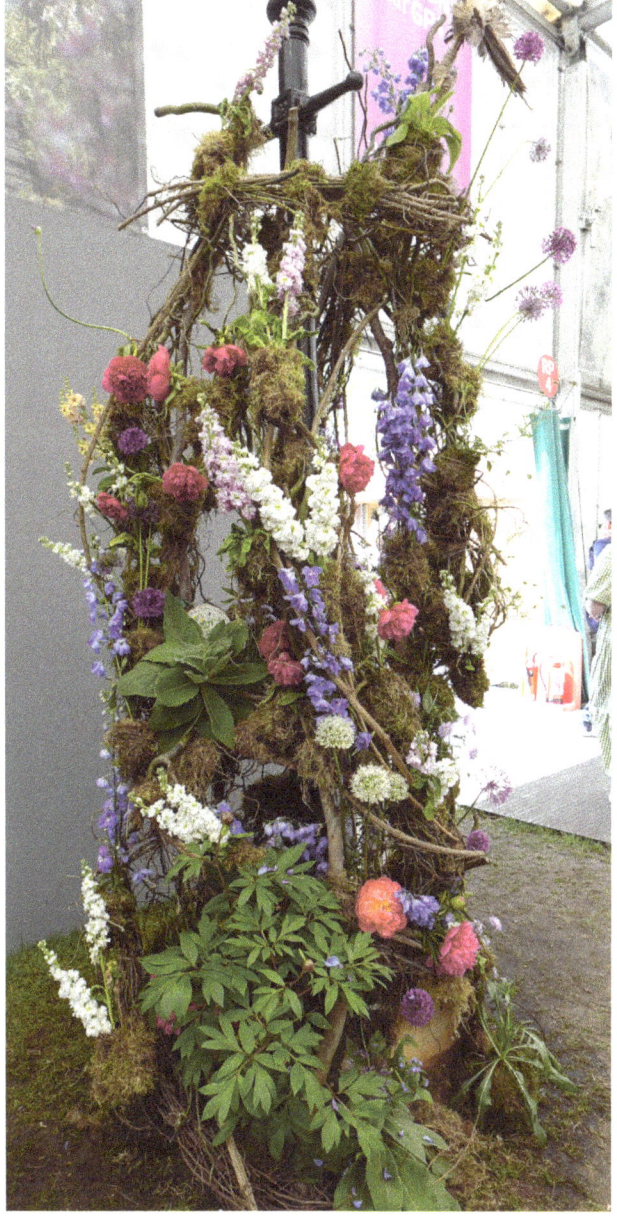

stocks in white and pink, and the blue delphinium, white allium, and the splendid colour of rose-coloured peony flowers, all make for an interesting combination within the visual experience.

The strength of the blocking of the green delphinium foliage gives a nice transition to the mossy base.

Like all floral designs shown, each one is an expression of the creator! Below, this 'Gold' winning design, titled, 'On The Verge,' has tall, elegant placements which add the necessary height to incorporate the lamppost, which is an accessory to the overall design.

The autumn colours incorporated in the lower placements add to the depth of creativity.

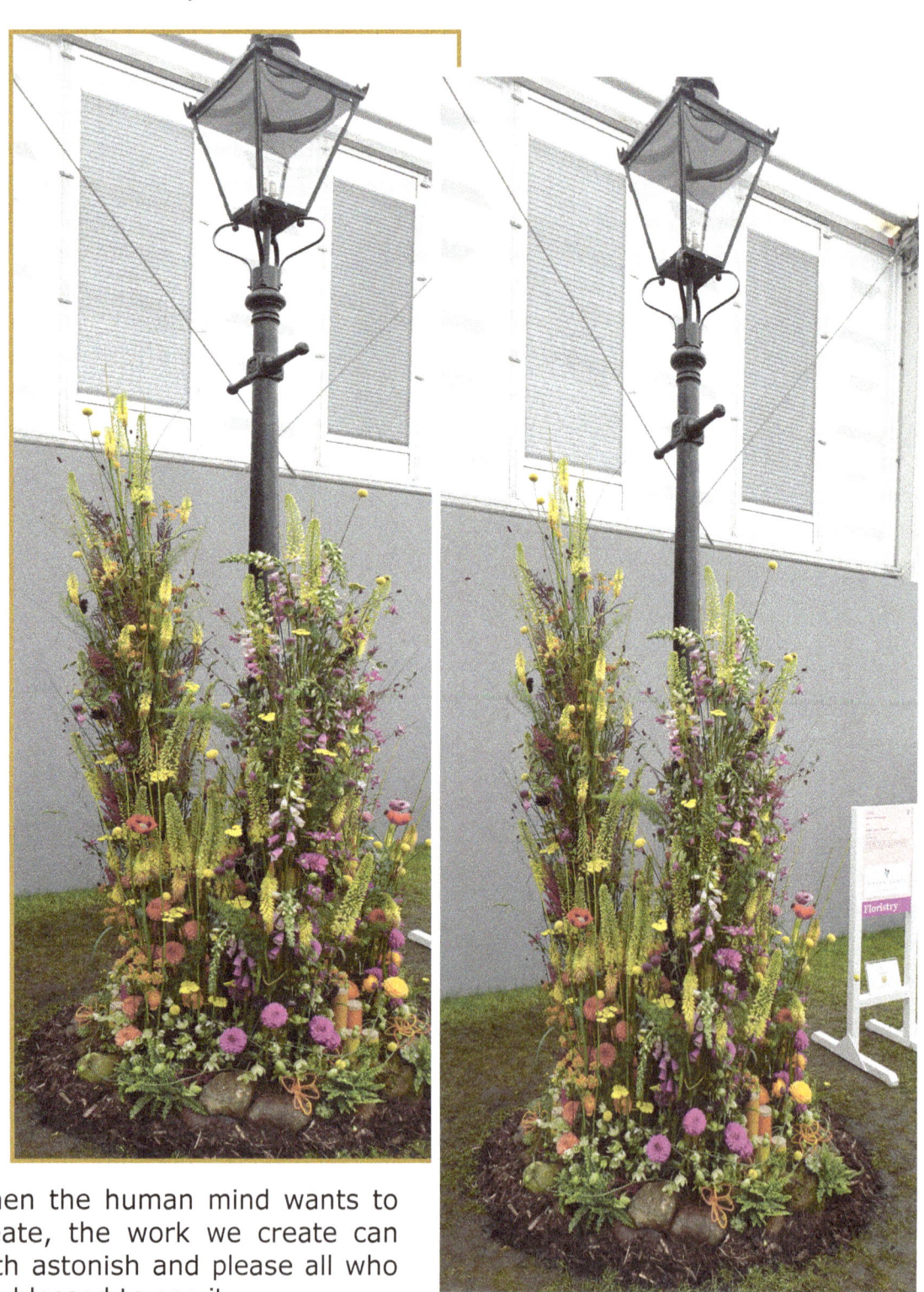

When the human mind wants to create, the work we create can both astonish and please all who are blessed to see it.

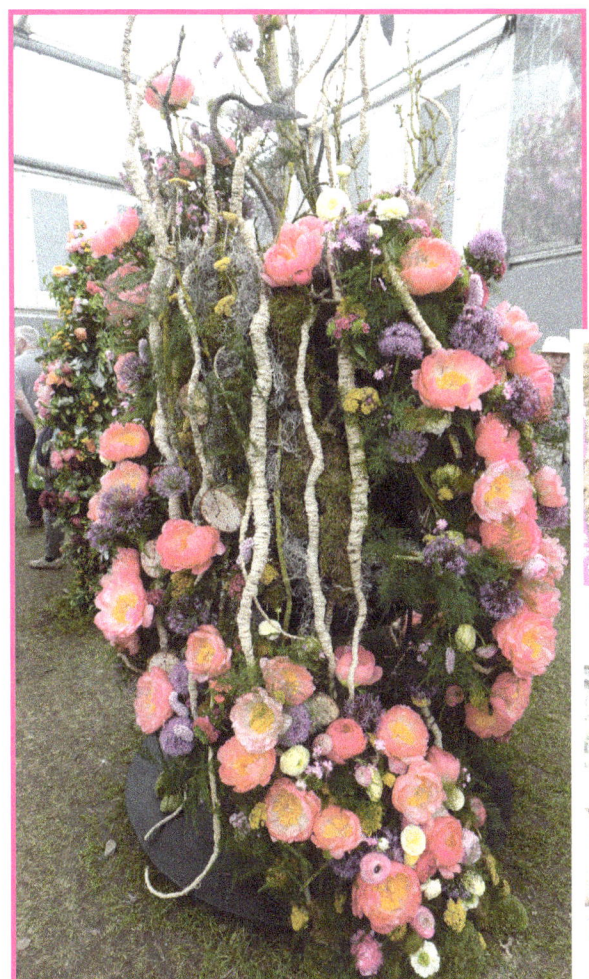

'Magnificent,' were the words I used when I first saw this wonderful, massed work. From the 'eye-catching' moment of seeing the double fern-leaf peony, the raffia wrapped twine threading its way through the design, and then looking deeply to the smaller placements of lavender to purple flowers, and again the use of the Hogarth Curve in the flowing lines; the overall combination was breathtaking.

When such magnificent blooms as the peony is grown to capture the visual impact of the spectator, we know within our hearts, that someone, somewhere, has worked very hard.

The appearance of a clock face on the different ends of sawn wood, help in the fun of the moment in the design. There are no sombre moments, just a time to look and enjoy the pleasure of the beauty before you.

The Magnificence of The Peony...

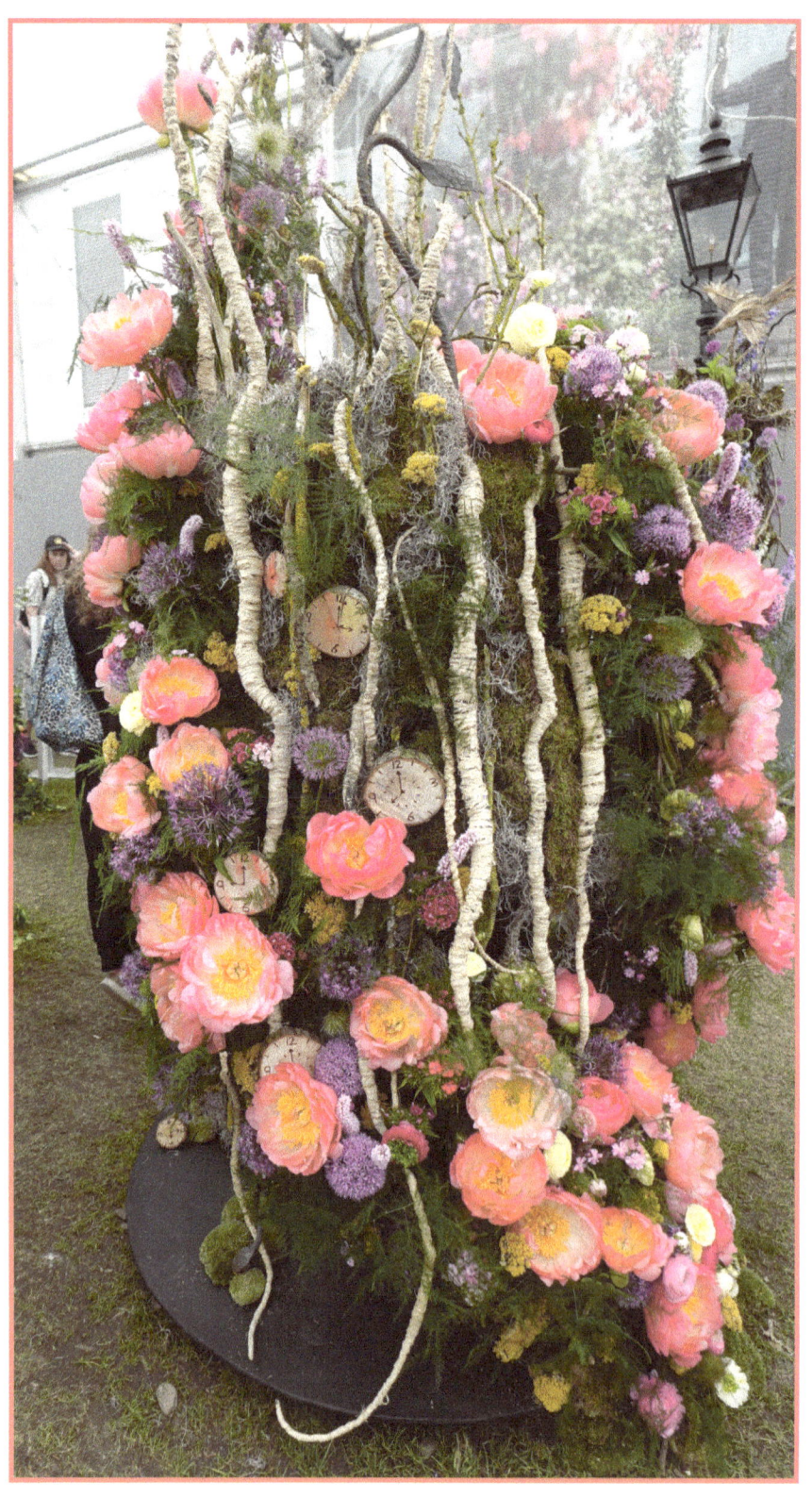

Floristry and Floral Art

Elegance and structure help to bring about this beautiful Ikebana design.

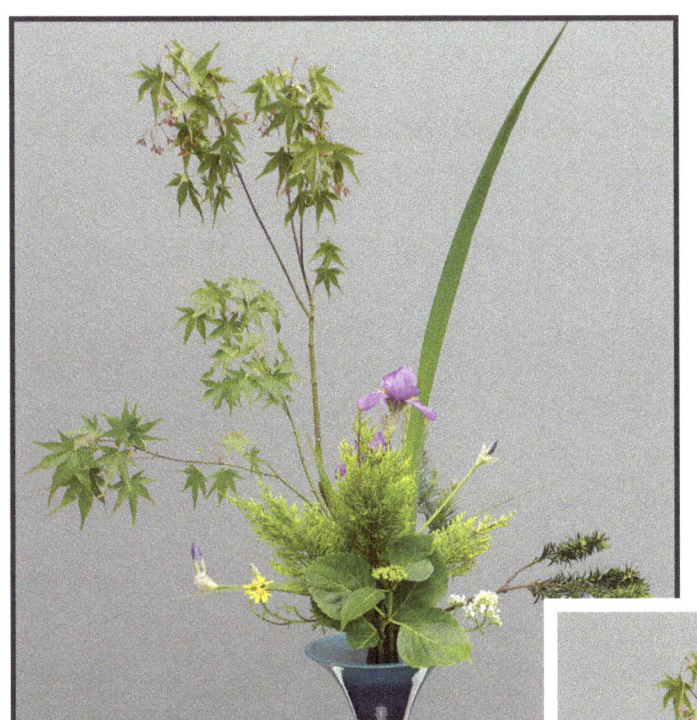

As part of my own journey into design, I spent a year attending weekly classes with an Ikebana Master artist in Australia. It was a beautiful time used in total creation and the absorption of the positive use of line, space, movement, and materials.

Each movement has meaning including earth, water, and sky.

The use of the new shoots within the maple branch placements, the strength of the line from what may be a gladiolus, sword shaped leaf, the use of a full flower iris and the iris buds, with a placement of hydrangea stem complete with new buds and fresh leaves, then the placement of one yellow wildflower daisy all adds to the rhythm of this design.

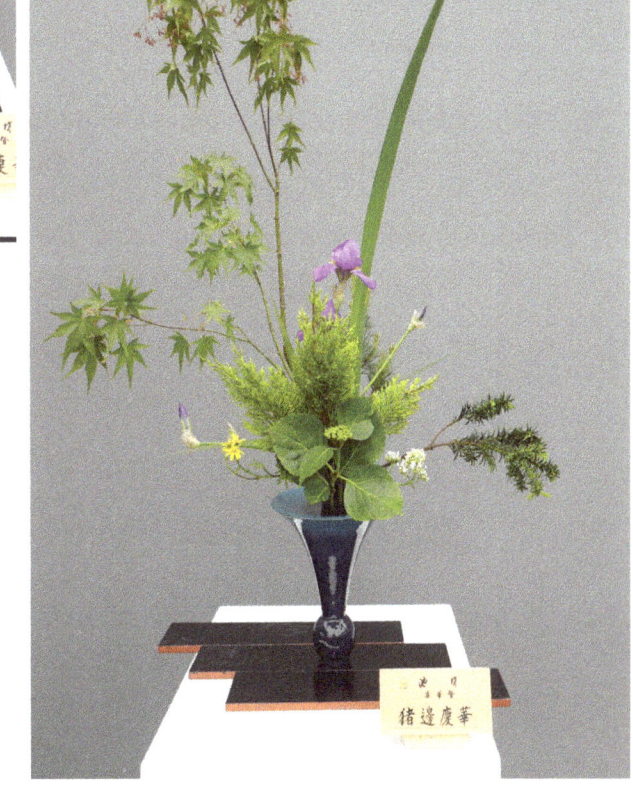

The Florist

Not knowing what to do, the time had come, to leave school and look for a trade and start the new…!

With no decisions formed, the mind was empty, and age did not understand, for if not a career chosen, the future will obscure from view…!

Urgency was emphasized and plans all set, an interview was made, 'But your parents' must attend' I was told…!

Not knowing what to expect, the interview over and new trade begun, and to begin, it was not much fun…!

Hard days were earnt, small wages were received; from thinking now… It was only three pounds a week and not a lot could be done…!

But learning was the 'call of the day,' for they had much to give, and much to say…!

Constance Spry, was a name often heard, and my teachers were brought in, for they were teachers of much renown…!

For hours were spent doing and learning, but filled with 'in-between time' were hard and cold, so much to do, long hours were spent…

Mossing wire frames, for many unnamed – funerals, I learnt a lot, dead people were a daily mention: work hard and do not relent…!

For this was an investment into the future and time well spent…!

Cold winter mornings, Christmas is near, holly wreaths to make, displays filled with ice, for this time was cold and not nice…!

Spring would come and daffodils appear, how lovely to see the bright smiling faces, and the very good cheer…!

Those sunny days of learning, the art, and the skill…, for those days have stood well with me, and I learnt to the fill…!

For the question I constantly asked of my mind: 'Why do people buy flowers…?'

For onto university, I needed to ask, which allowed me to research and discover for hours and hours…!

The reason people buy flowers is an emotional need…!
A sense of expression, a sense of happiness, of love, of sadness they may feel…!

And so it is, the florist's role, is not only about, beauty and creation…!

But about the need to give to another… And the need to give to that individual soul…!

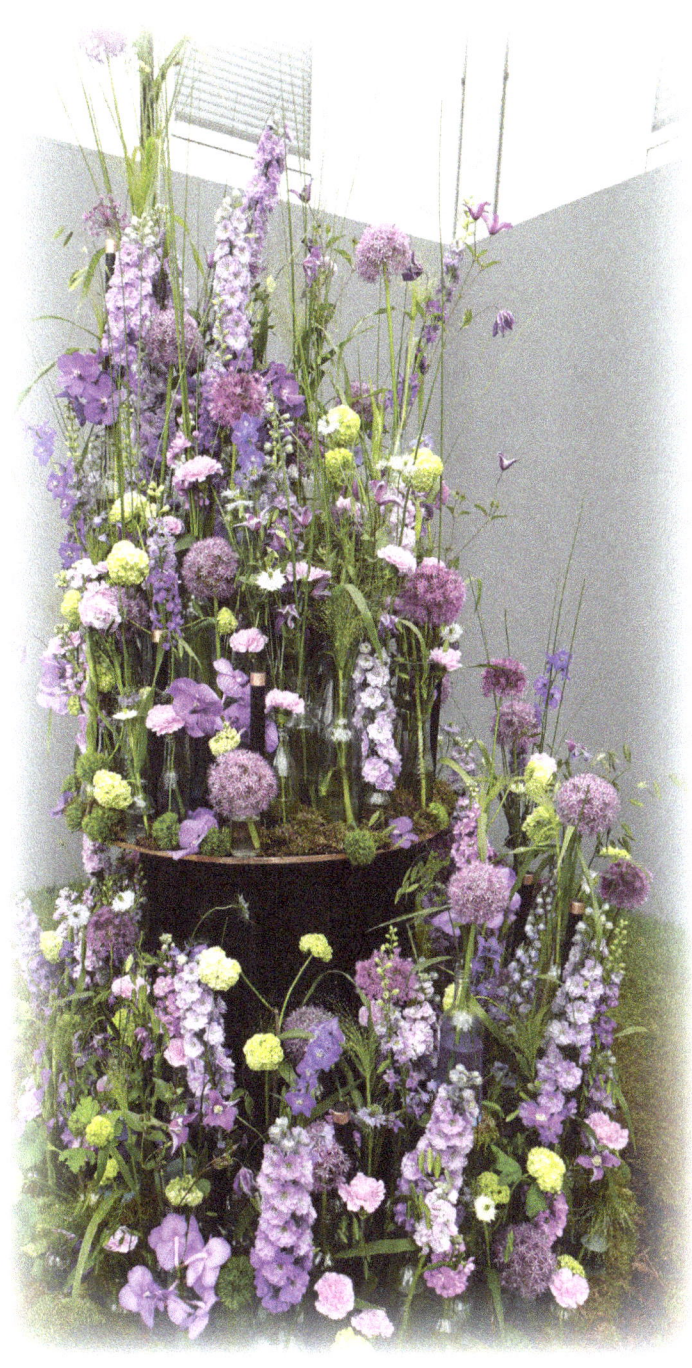

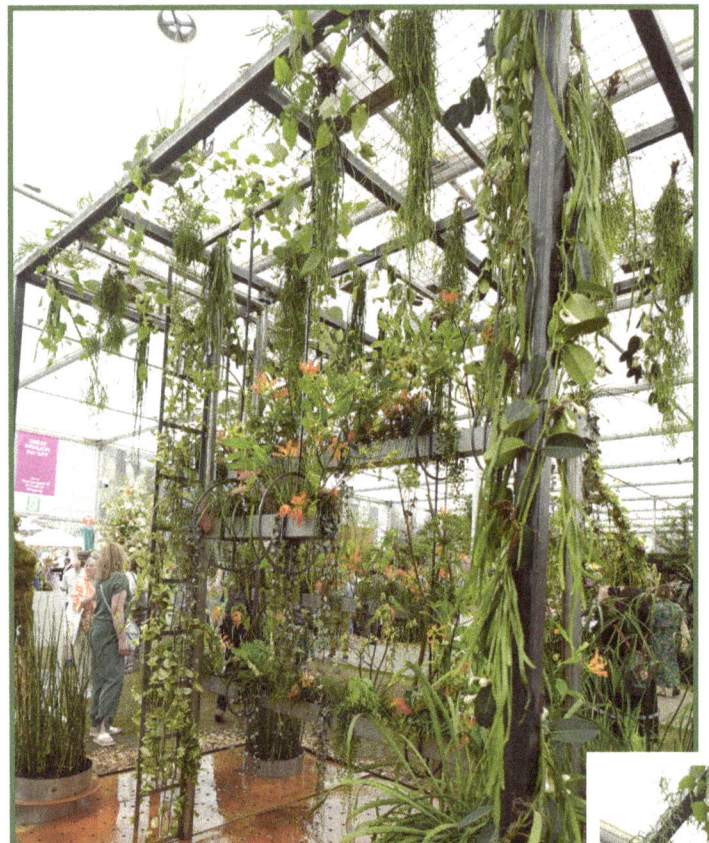

Opposite, this is not necessarily a flower arrangement, but it has a combination of elements that may allow it to fit into this position. Cool, refreshing and the use of foliage to create the feeling that you are within the rain forest of some magical land.

Interspersed within the green plant placements are small touches of the orange colour gloriosa lily and just at times a touch of white is added...!

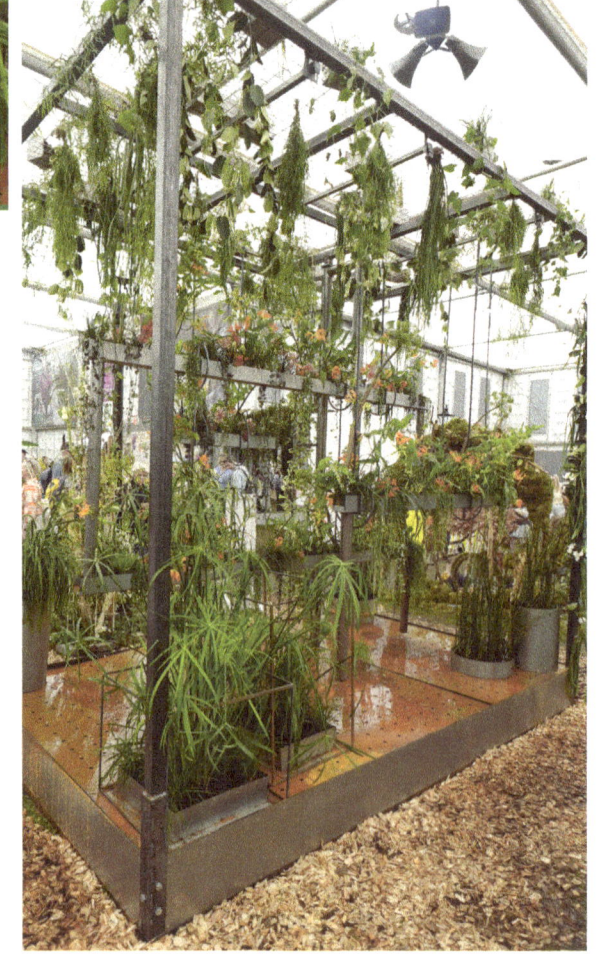

The grey square frame that acts as the boundaries within the design are strong in appearance when contrasted with the delicate placements of leaf and flower materials.

And then, the water is added to the base of the design supporting the resemblance to a rain forest of South America, some parts of Asia and of course, to Northern Australia, and other related areas that encourage natural growth in safe and clean environments.

The use of different mosses and occasionally the use of pink fungi, make this a masterful design.

The Mush Room

Mushrooms, mushrooms, mushrooms, what else is needed?

With so many, now edible varieties being produced, mushrooms not only look wonderful in many culinary delights, but they are good for the human body, and brain when incorporated into our everyday diet.

There are many benefits to the human body when mushrooms are in the food we eat. Mushrooms contain Riboflavin, which is good for our blood cell production, they also contain many of the B vitamins including niacin and pantothenic acid which help to support and protect the heart. Niacin helps to support our digestive systems and keeping our skin healthy.

Mushrooms also contain antioxidants which help to eliminate cancer.

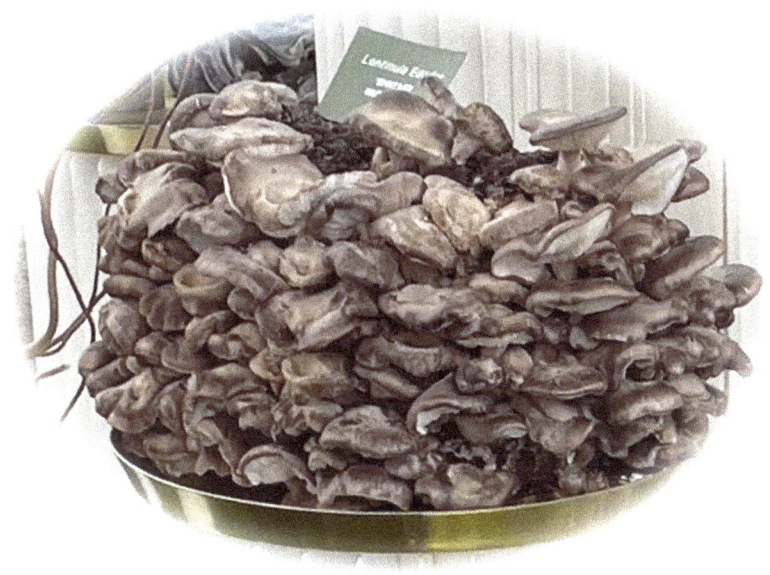

The Mush Room...

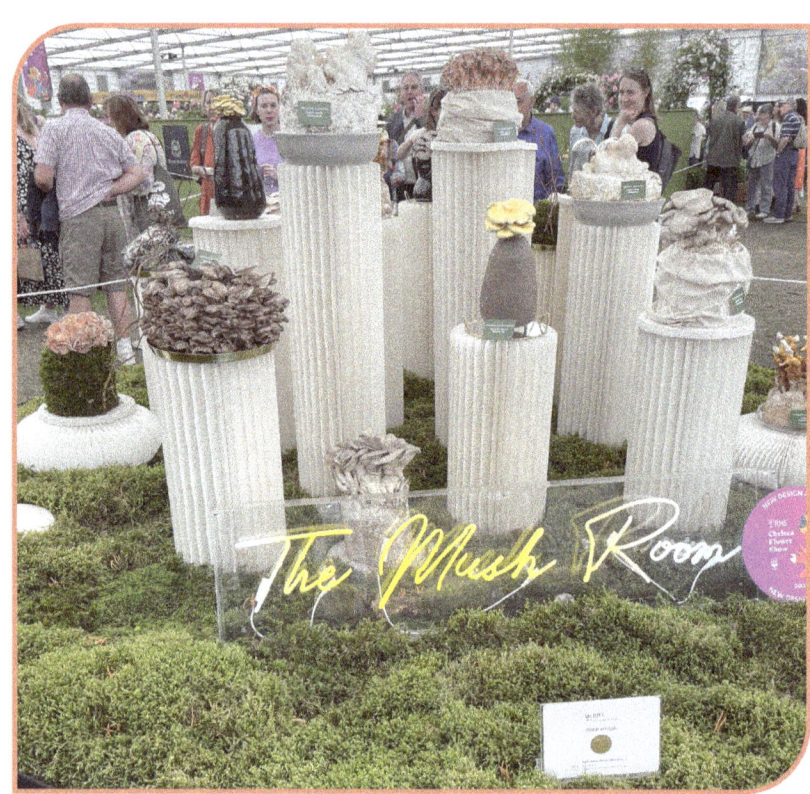

To say the minimum would not be enough. To at first see this stand with such a variety of different shaped and coloured mushrooms, was intriguing. The shapes, some of which, look like sculptures, were so different.

The natural development of nature's own artistic structures in the Design Elements have been used to the maximum extent.

The use of shape, colour, impact was at natures beck-and-call as the natural form of the mushrooms grew into shape.

From soft-rose pinks, to lemons, white, cream and more. Of course, not forgetting the familiar browns of the species.

Enhancing the shapes through tasteful and singular white stands, all of which mimicked the underside of many different groups of mushrooms.

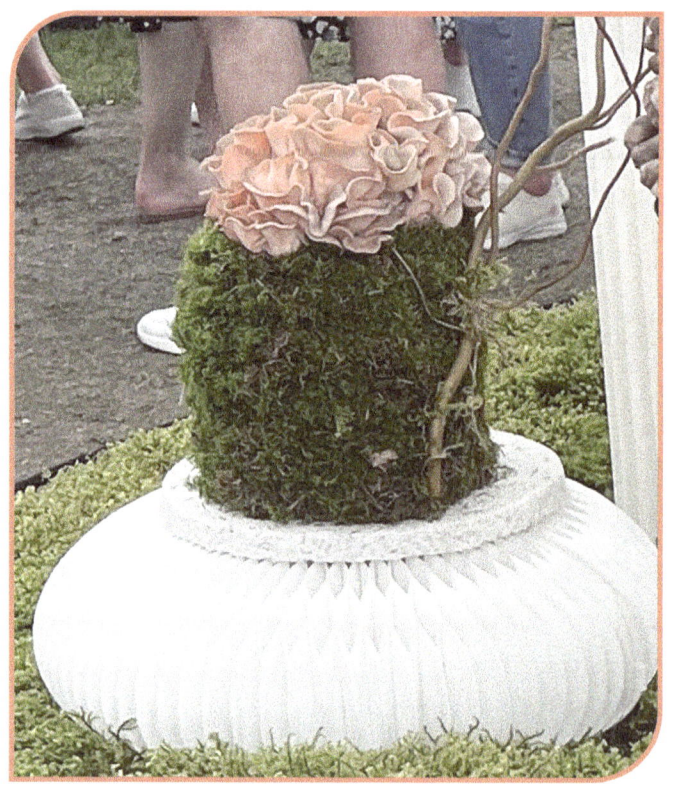

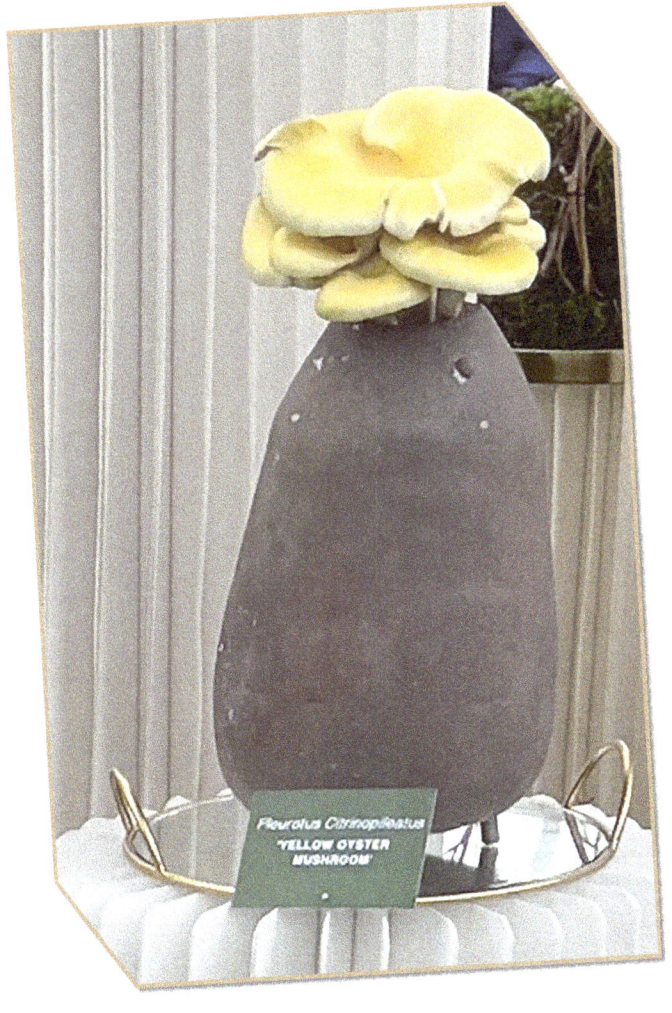

Opposite, this lemon oyster mushroom was outstanding as it stood in the display. The top of the traditional shaped mushroom, which most of us would be familiar with, is smooth, with the undulation seen on the underside! This mushroom is similar in appearance.

Not only do mushrooms offer many health benefits, but they can distinguish many culinary dishes which may be seen in restaurants and other good food outlets.

From lemons to the more familiar browns, (below). often seen in our supermarkets. These however, do look appear to grow from one solid-central structure, which may be wood or a moss-type base.

With so many mushrooms in the natural world, without the cultivated types now being developed, we may see an explosion of colours and shapes in the future.

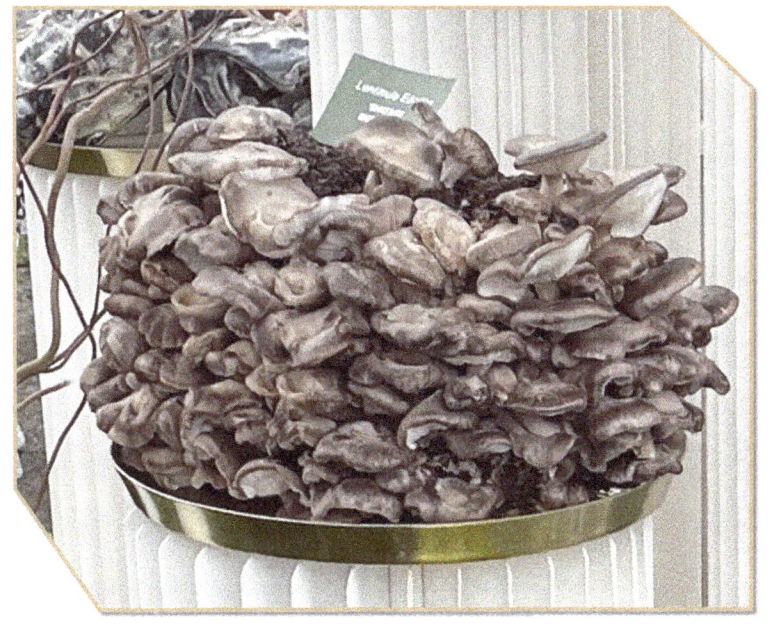

Shapes, Colour & Texture

The word 'Fascination...' comes to mind when we took the time to look closely at these different species of mushrooms.

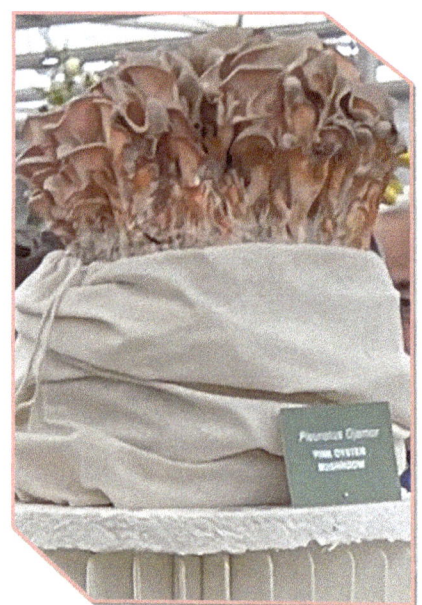

Each display makes a talking point, and each has its own story to tell.

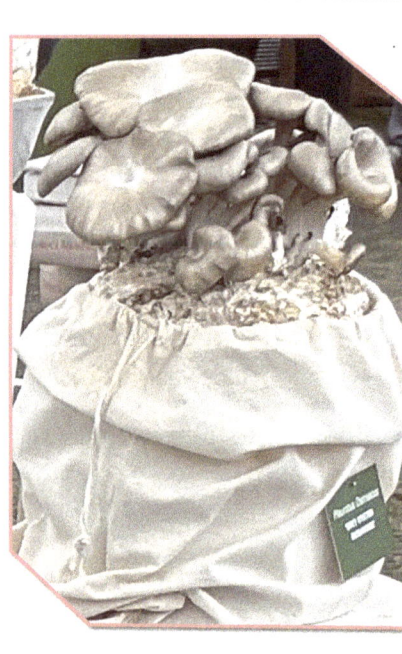

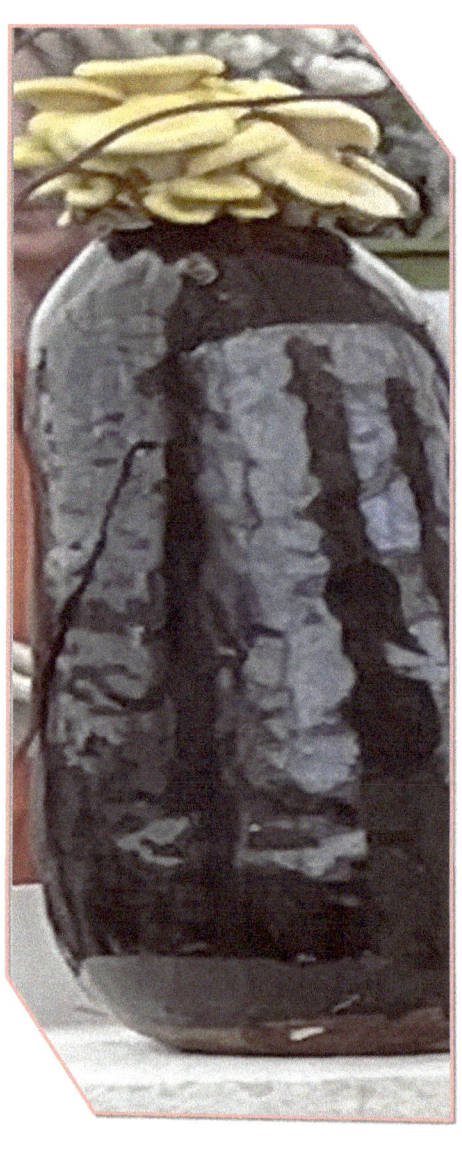

Caley Bros are taking the mushroom to new and enviable heights in the array of gourmet and medicinal, home-grown mushrooms.

All the mushroom displays sit on paper plinths. For growing nutrition of the plants, Caley Bros use coffee grounds, sawdust, soy hulls and old books. All are grown from waste products and can be readily grown at home.

We know you have enjoyed this special book,
Part 2 is now available at your local bookstore
or directly from

www.how2books.com.au

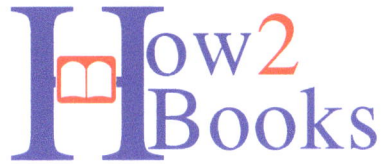

Other Books That May Interest You

Available Online
www.how2books.com.au

The book, 'How To Create Easy Wedding Bouquets', introduces you to many techniques in wedding bouquet construction, the different methods used to wire different flowers and leaves, how to tape, ribboning the wedding bouquet handle, how to make a corsage, buttonhole and other industry techniques that will start you on a floristry career.

Our education company, Full Potential Education And Training has been developed to support people who want to learn how to build skills for the floristry industry. The course is a CPD Accredited 20-week online course in commercial floristry wedding bouquet making. It has been designed to support people who want to work for themselves and start a business or for those people who want a trade career in the floristry industry. For more information, please email, admin@fullpotentialtraining.com.au

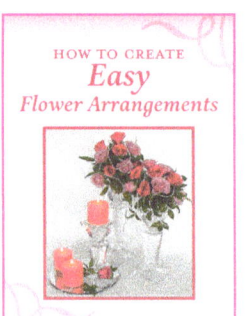

The book, 'How To Create Easy Flower Arrangements', is an introduction to floral art and commercial floristry in flower arranging. The book is designed to help those people who want to learn flower arranging and construction techniques and will give the foundation knowledge to those people who want to work in the floristry industry.

It will also help people who want to learn flower arranging for pleasure and gift giving, and those people who create flower arrangements for special occasions.

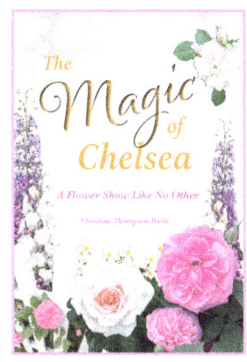
The Magic of Chelsea, 2022, is full of information covering the Chelsea Flower Show, floristry, art and design, sculpture, different plants and how they are used and has other informative and relevant information that gives the reader different information about the topics included. It would be an ideal book for florists, garden centres, nurseries and like businesses to have as a book for sale in their business. For wholesale information, please email: admin@booksforreadingonline.com

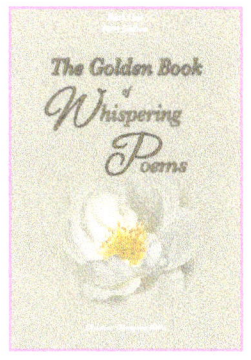
Because we love the books we create, and poetry is a big part of the work we do, we could not help ourselves but include this book of different poetry.

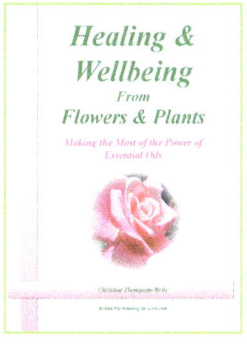
Without plants, we cannot survive. As all flower and lovers know, many plants and trees are under threat! Plants not only help to keep our planet and wildlife healthy, but they also add to our human wellbeing.

This book outlines the benefits of using herbs in our everyday lives. It is colourful and gives a breakdown of herb uses.

All the books are available at
www.how2books.com.au
This book is brought to you from the publishers of:

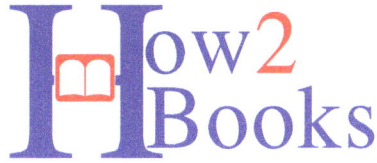

ISBN: 978-0-6459403-6-7

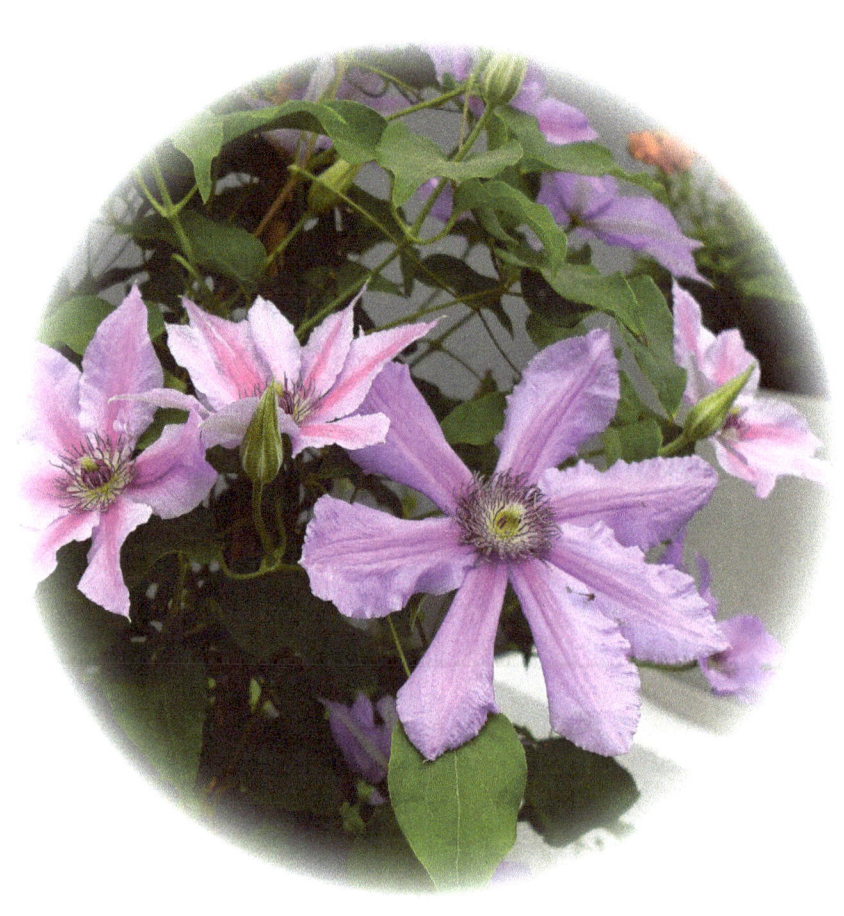

www.ingramcontent.com/pod-product-compliance
Lightning Source LLC
Chambersburg PA
CBHW041711290426
44109CB00028B/2847